Antibody Therapy

THE MEDICAL PERSPECTIVES SERIES

Advisors:

David Hames *Department of Biochemistry and Molecular Biology, University of Leeds, Leeds, U.K.*

David R. Harper *Department of Virology, Medical College of St Bartholomew's Hospital, London, U.K.*

Andrew P. Read *Department of Medical Genetics, University of Manchester, Manchester, U.K.*

Robin Winter *Institute of Child Health, London, U.K.*

Oncogenes and Tumor Suppressor Genes
Cytokines
The Human Genome
Autoimmunity
Genetic Engineering
Asthma
DNA Fingerprinting
Molecular Virology
HIV and AIDS
Human Vaccines and Vaccination
Antibody Therapy

Forthcoming titles:

Antimicrobial Drug Action
Antiviral Therapy

Antibody Therapy

Edward J. Wawrzynczak
Rothschild Bioscience Unit, Five Arrows House, St Swithin's Lane,
London EC4N 8NR

© **BIOS Scientific Publishers Limited, 1995**

First published 1995

A CIP catalogue record for this book is available from the British Library.

ISBN 1 872748 29 5

BIOS Scientific Publishers Ltd
9 Newtec Place, Magdalen Road, Oxford OX4 1RE, UK
Tel. +44 (0)1865 726286. Fax +44 (0)1865 246823

DISTRIBUTORS

Australia and New Zealand
    DA Information Services
    648 Whitehorse Road, Mitcham
    Victoria 3132

Singapore and South East Asia
    Toppan Company (S) PTE Ltd
    38 Liu Fang Road, Jurong
    Singapore 2262

India
    Viva Books Private Limited
    4325/3 Ansari Road, Daryaganj
    New Delhi 110 002

USA and Canada
    Books International Inc.
    PO Box 605, Herndon, VA 22070

Typeset by Footnote Graphics, Warminster, Wilts, UK.
Printed by Information Press Ltd, Oxford, UK.

Contents

Abbreviations

aa	amino acid
ADCC	antibody-dependent cellular cytotoxicity
ADEPT	antibody-directed enzyme prodrug therapy
AIDS	acquired immune deficiency syndrome
ALG	anti-lymphocyte globulin
APC	antigen-presenting cell
Asn	asparagine
ATG	anti-thymocyte globulin
bFGF	basic fibroblast growth factor
bmt	bone marrow transplantation
C	constant (gene, domain or region)
CD	cluster of differentiation (antigen)
CDR	complementarity-determining region
CEA	carcino embryonic antigen
CMV	cytomegalovirus
CSF	colony-stimulating factor
CTL	cytotoxic T lymphocyte
Cys	cysteine
D	diversity (gene)
EBV	Epstein–Barr virus
EGF	epidermal growth factor
EMA	epithelial membrane antigen
Fab	antigen-binding fragment
Fc	crystallizable fragment
FR	framework region
Fv	variable region fragment
G-CSF	granulocyte-colony stimulating factor
GI	gastrointestinal
GM-CSF	granulocyte/macrophage-colony stimulating factor
GVHD	graft-versus-host disease
H	heavy (chain)
HAMA	human anti-mouse antibody

HBV	hepatitis B virus
HCV	hepatitis C virus
HIV	human immunodeficiency virus
HMW-MAA	high molecular weight melanoma-associated antigen
HR	hypervariable region
HSV	herpes simplex virus
id	idiotype
im	intramuscular
ip	intraperitoneal
iv	intravenous
IFN	interferon
Ig	immunoglobulin
IL	interleukin
ITP	idiopathic thrombocytopenic purpura
IVIG	intravenous immunoglobulin
J	joining (gene)
L	light (chain)
Lys	lysine
Mab	monoclonal antibody
MHC	major histocompatibility complex
MI	myocardial infarction
NK	natural killer (cell)
PAF	platelet-activating factor
PEM	polymorphic epithelial mucin
PTCA	percutaneous translumenal coronary angioplasty
RAID	radioimmunodiagnosis
RAIT	radioimmunotherapy
RES	reticuloendothelial system
RhD	Rhesus D (antigen)
RIGS	radioimmunoguided surgery
RSV	respiratory syncytial virus
sc	subcutaneous
sdm	site-directed mutagenesis
SCID	severe combined immunodeficiency disease
SIRS	systemic inflammatory response syndrome
TAA	tumor-associated antigen
TCR	T cell receptor
TNF	tumor necrosis factor
Tyr	tyrosine
V	variable (gene, domain or region)
VEGF	vascular endothelial growth factor
VZV	varicella zoster virus
wt	wild-type

Preface

Antibody therapy developed as a major interest of mine during several highly enjoyable years of active research. At the same time, I was privileged to lecture on this topic to students attending a number of immunology courses and summer schools. A source of frustration was the superficial, out-of-date or inaccurate treatment frequently afforded antibody therapy in textbooks despite the central importance of antibodies in immunology. The impetus for writing this book stemmed in large part from the desire to remedy this deficiency.

My intention has been to provide a systematic and comprehensive review of antibody therapy in a single volume. I have tried to strike a balance between that which is important and well-established, and that which is interesting or innovative though may not be easily turned into practice. My hope is that the book will serve both as a useful introduction to the area and as a guide to understanding both the state-of-the-art and future developments. Ultimately, the content and the emphasis are my responsibility as indeed are any failings.

Thanks are due to Dr Jonathan Ray and his colleagues at BIOS for their patient and professional guidance and to Dr David Harper for his constructive advice during the writing of the book. I am also grateful to Professor Herman Waldmann for suggesting a number of improvements in style and content. Finally, the time spent in writing this book was lost elsewhere: I am indebted to Anne, Robert and Toby for their understanding and support.

E. J. Wawrzynczak, Ph.D.

Chapter 1

Structure and function of antibodies

1.1 Introduction

The immune system acts to protect the body against infection by micro-organisms, such as viruses and bacteria, and against the harmful effects of noninfectious foreign substances. Immunity is constituted by a number of specific and nonspecific defense mechanisms that include physical barriers to the entry of foreign agents, immune cells in the blood and tissues, and macromolecules in the circulation. Specific immunity is coordinated by multiple elements of the immune system and is classified into two different systems. The cellular immune response involves cells called T lymphocytes that are present in the blood and tissues and act to eliminate microbial invaders directly. The humoral immune response involves macromolecules called antibodies that are found in the blood and tissues and in secretory fluids. Antibodies, or immunoglobulins (Igs), are soluble globular proteins that bind selectively to foreign substances and stimulate protective immune effector mechanisms as a consequence of binding. The properties of the humoral immune response are shaped by the genetics, development and physiology of the B lymphocyte cells that make antibodies. The molecular and biological characteristics of antibody molecules, which have evolved to play a key role in the action of the body's immune defense system, form the basis for their use in the prophylaxis and therapy of human disease.

1.2 The humoral immune response

1.2.1 Antigens and immunogens

An antigen is a molecule that interacts with an antibody. Most types of macromolecule including proteins, nucleic acids, polysaccharides and lipids can be antigens. An antigen that is capable of inducing an active specific immune response is called an immunogen. In general, only macromolecules that are foreign to an animal will stimulate an immune response. Small natural or synthetic molecules can also induce an immune response in an animal provided that the antigen is linked to an

1

immunogenic macromolecule. The small molecule is commonly known as the hapten and the macromolecule, usually a protein, is called the carrier. A large immunogenic molecule may encompass a number of different structures, known as antigenic determinants or epitopes, that are capable of being recognized independently by the immune system. In proteins, epitopes may be linear determinants that are formed by adjacent amino acid (aa) residues from a continuous portion of the polypeptide backbone. Alternatively, protein epitopes may be complex conformational or discontinuous determinants that are formed by aa residues from different regions of the primary structure that are juxtaposed by the three-dimensional folding of the polypeptide. A macromolecule that contains repetitive structures may display multiple identical antigenic determinants.

1.2.2 Antibody–antigen interaction

Antibody molecules interact with antigen to form reversible noncovalent complexes. Binding depends upon complementarity between the structures of the antigen and the antigen-combining site of the antibody. The strength of interaction between an antigen and the complementary antigen-combining site of an antibody, which can be measured as an association or dissociation constant, is known as the affinity. Natural antibodies are Y-shaped molecules that contain two antigen-combining sites (Section 1.3). Bivalent antibodies may attach by both antigen-combining sites to a macromolecule that contains multiple antigenic determinants or to a cell or virus that displays an array of identical antigen molecules on its surface. The overall strength of antibody binding is then known as the avidity. An antibody with two antigen-combining sites of comparatively low affinity for antigen may none the less bind tightly to a multimeric antigen because the combination of low-affinity interactions results in high avidity. Polymeric antibody molecules with more than two antigen-combining sites demonstrate even higher binding avidity. Alternatively, antibodies can cross-link multimeric antigens to form immune complexes that comprise a lattice of antibody–antigen interactions.

1.2.3 Immunization

The immune system has the capacity to generate large numbers of antibodies in response to exposure to an immunogen, a process called immunization. When primed by immunization, the immune system of an animal responds by making a diverse range of antibodies with structurally distinct antigen-combining sites. The primary immune response to an initial exposure to antigen generates antibodies directed against different antigenic determinants and antibodies that recognize similar epitopes yet have structurally distinct antigen-combining sites. A subsequent repeat exposure to a specific antigen typically gives rise to a secondary antibody response that is both more rapid and of greater magnitude than that triggered by the first exposure. In addition, the humoral response to a particular antigen alters qualitatively with time and results in the production of antibodies with enhanced antigen-recognition properties. The antibody response is self-regulating, being subject to feedback-control mechanisms that act to limit the extent of antigen-specific responses. Moreover, the response is controlled to prevent the generation of antibodies able to react destructively with the animal's own, or 'self', antigens (Sections 1.4 and 1.5).

1.3 Antibody structure

1.3.1 Immunoglobulin structure

Antibody molecules have specialized functions determined by their structure, although different types of antibody have a broadly similar overall structure. The basic Ig molecule is a Y-shaped molecule in which different functions are localized in discrete parts of the molecule (*Figure 1.1*). The antigen-combining sites of the antibody are located in the regions that form the tips of the two identical Fab arms of the molecule. The region that forms the stem of the antibody molecule, the Fc region, is principally responsible for interactions with other components of the immune system (Section 1.6). The Fab arms are linked to the Fc region by a flexible hinge region. The Ig molecule is made up of four polypeptide chains: two identical heavy (H) chains and two identical light (L) chains.

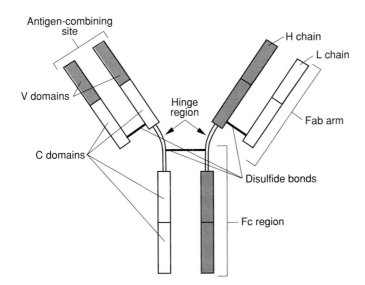

Figure 1.1: Structure of immunoglobulin molecules.

The two H chains associate with each other and each H chain also associates with a single L chain. Chain association occurs through strong noncovalent interactions and the H–H and H–L chain pairs are also linked covalently by one or more inter-chain disulfide bonds, depending on the antibody type. Ig chains are formed of repeating units of a homologous structure, of about 110 aa residues, that folds independently into a compact domain known as the Ig-fold. The basic Ig domain consists of two layers of β-pleated sheet, each made up of three or four strands of anti-parallel polypeptide chain, that pack together to form a roughly cylindrical sandwich-like structure with a hydrophobic interior and with loops exposed at the ends of the strands. The two β-pleated sheets are linked by a single internal intra-chain disulfide bond located close to the center of the domain.

1.3.2 Antibody variable domains

The aa sequences of H and L chains from different antibodies are more diverse in the amino-terminal Ig domains, denoted the variable (V) domains, than in the carboxy-terminal Ig domains known as the constant (C) domains (*Figure 1.1*). In fact, V domains contain stretches of relatively conserved aa sequence, called framework regions (FRs), interspersed with regions that display considerable aa sequence variability between antibodies recognizing different antigens, known as hypervariable regions (HRs). V domains follow the structure of the basic Ig-fold, although they possess an extra two strands in one β-sheet and an additional loop that connects these strands when compared with the C domains (*Figure 1.2*). The three HRs of aa sequence in each chain correspond with polypeptide loops that connect β-strands at the top of the V domain. The HR loops are involved in forming the antigen-combining site and so are also known as complementarity-determining regions (CDRs). Although HRs show wide variability in aa sequence, there are similarities in structure between different CDR loops. A limited repertoire of preferred polypeptide chain conformations, referred to as canonical structures, have been identified for HR1, HR2 and HR3 of the L chain, and HR1 and HR2 of the H chain. A number of CDR loops incorporate a reverse-turn structure dictated by the presence of particular aa residues that have favored H-bonding, packing or torsional orientations in key positions. The HR3 of the H chain is characterized by much greater diversity in terms of length, aa sequence and conformation (Section 1.5).

1.3.3 The antigen-combining site

The more highly conserved FRs of the V domains are very similar in antibodies of the same type. The aa sequence of the FRs determines the

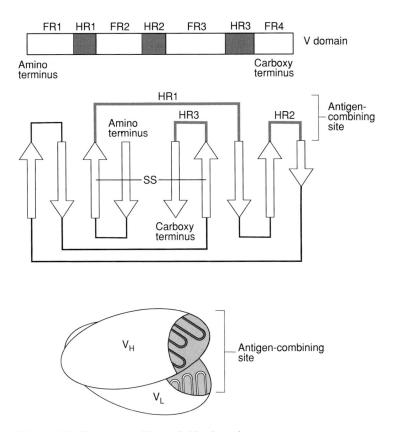

Figure 1.2: Structure of Ig variable domains.

three-dimensional fold of the V domain, the display of the antigen-binding CDR loops and the interaction between the V domains of the H and L chains, denoted V_H and V_L, respectively. Within each Fab arm of the antibody, the V_H and V_L domains associate noncovalently because of structural complementarity between conserved aa residues present at the hydrophobic interface between the two domains. The association of the V_H and V_L domains positions the three CDRs from each chain in close proximity and determines their precise conformation in the antigen-combining site. The cluster of CDR loops creates a cleft or contoured pocket with a relatively large surface available to interact with antigen by multiple electrostatic, H-bonding, van der Waals and hydrophobic interactions (*Figure 1.3*). The spatial distribution of the CDR aa residues in the combining site principally determines the antigen-binding characteristics of an antibody molecule. The CDRs present in the antigen-combining site contribute to the affinity of antigen

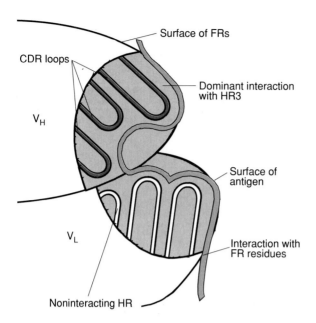

Figure 1.3: Antigen binding in the combining site of antibody (schematic representation).

binding to different extents depending upon the structure of the antigen. In general, the CDRs of the H chain, and HR3 in particular, are prominent in antigen binding. However, not all the CDRs of the V_H and V_L domains necessarily participate in antigen binding, especially when the antigen is a small molecule. The structure of the FRs determines the precise conformation of the CDR loops and thus indirectly influences antigen binding. In addition, FR aa residues may be involved in direct contact with the antigen in the combining site of the antibody.

1.3.4 Structure of IgG

Immunoglobulin G, or IgG (150 kDa approx.), is the major class or isotype of Ig in the blood of mammals and is the principal type of antibody produced in the secondary immune response. IgG consists of two H chains (50 kDa approx.) and two L chains (25 kDa approx.) (*Figure 1.4*). The H chain comprises a V_H domain and a C region that consists of three Ig domains denoted C_H1, C_H2 and C_H3. The L chain consists of a V_L domain and a single C domain called C_L. The V_L and C_L domains of one L chain associate noncovalently with the V_H and C_H1 domains of one H chain, respectively, to form an Fab arm. The C_H2 and C_H3 domains of the two H chains also interact together to form the Fc region of the antibody. Strong hydrophobic interactions occur between the two C_H3

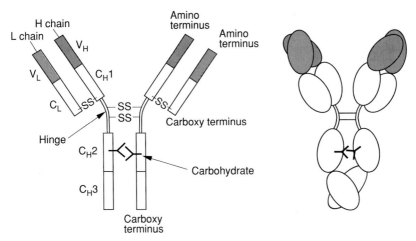

Figure 1.4: Structure of human IgG1.

domains. The C_H2 domains do not engage in extensive protein–protein contacts that are typical of other domains in intact IgG. Instead, oligosaccharide side-chains, located in the region between the C_H2 domains of each H chain (Section 1.3.6), form the only physical contact. The hinge region between the C_H1 and C_H2 domains of the H chain is an extended nonglobular portion of the polypeptide backbone that allows flexibility of the Fab arms and Fc region relative to one another. The hinge contains the cysteine (Cys) residues which form the inter-chain disulfide bonds that covalently link the two H-chains together.

In humans, the IgG class of antibody can be subdivided into four IgG subclasses with homologous aa sequence, called IgG1, IgG2, IgG3 and IgG4, which incorporate γ1, γ2, γ3 and γ4 H-chain types respectively. Human IgG1 and IgG4 contain two inter-chain disulfide linkages in the hinge region, whereas IgG2 has four disulfide linkages. Human IgG3 contains an extended hinge region that appears to be a quadruplication of an IgG1-like hinge region. IgG1 is unique in the arrangement of its H–L chain linkage. The conserved Cys residue near the carboxy termi-nus of the L chain is disulfide bonded to an H chain Cys residue located between the $C_γ1$ and $C_γ2$ domains rather than between the V_H and $C_γ1$ domains, which is typical of other IgGs.

1.3.5 Structures of Ig classes

Ig classes are defined according to the kind of H chain that the antibody molecule contains. There are five major types of H chain – γ, μ, α, ε, and δ – that make up the five antibody classes IgG, IgM, IgA, IgE and IgD, respectively. Each type of H chain has a characteristic organization of Ig domains (*Figure 1.5*), whose structure determines the physiological

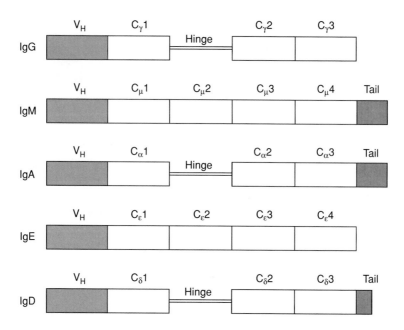

Figure 1.5: The domain structure of human Ig classes.

characteristics of the Ig class (Section 1.6). In each class of antibody, the H chain is associated with one of two types of L chain, either κ or λ.

IgM. IgM is the first type of antibody produced by the humoral immune response. The IgM molecule is a pentamer of Ig molecules (970 kDa approx.) that consist of two μ chains and two L chains. The μ chain comprises a V_H domain and a C region of four domains, C_H1, C_H2, C_H3 and C_H4, in which paired $C_\mu2$ domains are present instead of the hinge of IgG and the $C_\mu3$ and $C_\mu4$ domains resemble the $C_\gamma2$ and $C_\gamma3$ domains. The μ chain contains an additional short carboxy-terminal tail-piece that attaches to a joining chain responsible for pentamer formation.

IgA. IgA is the principal antibody type present in the mucous secretions of the gastrointestinal (GI) and respiratory tracts and breast milk. In the circulation, IgA exists predominantly in monomeric form (160 kDa approx.). In humans, there are two subclasses of IgA, called IgA1 and IgA2, that broadly resemble the structure of IgG. However, the $C_\alpha2$ domain forms additional disulfide bonds and lacks the equivalent of the carbohydrate chain present in the $C_\gamma2$ domain. The secretory form of IgA predominantly consists of a dimer of IgA monomers (350 kDa approx.) linked through an α chain tail-piece via a joining chain and a secretory component that forms part of the receptor responsible for the transepithelial transport of IgA to the mucosal surface.

IgE. IgE antibody is present at low levels bound tightly to receptors on mast cells that form part of the immune defense against certain pathogens. The ε chain of IgE, like IgM, has a C region with four domains. Uniquely, IgE (180 kDa approx.) contains disulfide bonds between the H chains at two positions, between the $C_\varepsilon 1$ and $C_\varepsilon 2$ domains, and between the $C_\varepsilon 2$ and $C_\varepsilon 3$ domains.

IgD. IgD (180 kDa approx.) resembles IgG except for a greatly extended hinge region and a short tail-piece. IgD is present in serum only at low levels and its function is unclear.

Cell-bound forms of IgM and IgD, which are present on the surface of B lymphocytes (Section 1.4.2), bear carboxy-terminal extensions that form additional transmembrane anchor sequences.

1.3.6 Antibody glycosylation

Antibody molecules are glycosylated in their C regions at characteristic positions determined by their isotype. The presence of carbohydrate influences the structure and physiological properties of Ig molecules (Section 1.6). In IgG, the carbohydrate is attached to an asparagine (Asn) residue at a unique site of glycosylation in the $C_\gamma 2$ domain. The oligosaccharide side-chains in the $C_\gamma 2$ domains are not of a single type but consist of a set of branched complex-type structures based on a mannosyl chitobiose core. The pattern of oligosaccharide side-chain heterogeneity is species-specific. IgM, IgE and IgD have interposed Asn-linked oligosaccharide side-chains in the equivalent domains to the $C_\gamma 2$ domains. IgM and IgE molecules possess additional carbohydrate in the $C_H 1$, $C_H 2$ and $C_H 3$ domains. The tail-pieces of IgM and IgA are also glycosylated. The principal difference between IgA1 and IgA2 is the structure of the hinge; IgA1 has a hinge region with five *O*-linked oligosaccharide side-chains in each α chain. Ig molecules can possess potential sites of carbohydrate addition in the V region, although such sites are not necessarily glycosylated in the native antibody molecule. The presence of oligosaccharide side-chains in the Fab arms can influence the antigen-binding characteristics of an antibody molecule.

1.3.7 Antibodies as antigens

Antibodies are complex glycoproteins that can be immunogenic in their own right. The specificity of immune responses serves to define structural differences between the various types of antibody. When an animal is immunized with xenogeneic Ig derived from another species, the antibody response that it generates is directed predominantly against epitopes present within the C domains of the H and L chains and can distinguish between isotypes that contain multiple differences in aa sequence. The antibody response is more restricted when an animal is immunized with Ig molecules from another individual of the same species. In this case, the antibodies induced detect minor differences between the aa sequences of C domains that reflect allelic polymorphisms. The antigenic structures are called allotypic determinants and antibody molecules with the same determinants are said to share the same allotype. Antigenic differences attributable to the unique structural features of the V domains are called idiotypic determinants, or idiotopes. Antibodies that express the same idiotopes are said to have cross-reacting, or 'public' idiotypes whereas antibodies expressing unique idiotopes have 'private' idiotypes.

1.4 The cellular basis of the antibody response

1.4.1 Immune-cell maturation

The cells of the immune system originate from a common progenitor, or stem cell, that resides in the bone marrow and is self-renewing during the individual's lifetime. Stem cells are pluripotent progenitor cells that differentiate into more specialized precursor cells and develop along different lineages to form mature immune cells during the process of hematopoiesis, or blood cell formation (*Table 1.1*). The maturation of blood cells along different lineages is regulated by a network of small, soluble proteins called interleukins (ILs) and colony-stimulating factors (CSFs), and known collectively as cytokines, that stimulate progenitor cells by binding to cell-surface receptors (*Table 1.2*).

Leukocytes are the white cells in the blood. Lymphocytes are the blood cells that are primarily responsible for antigen-specific immune responses. B lymphocytes, or B cells, synthesize and secrete antibody (Section 1.4.2). T lymphocytes, or T cells, have several roles: they mediate cellular immune responses, stimulate B cells to produce antibody and regulate the immune response (Sections 1.4.3–1.4.6). Monocytes in the blood and macrophages in the tissues play a critical role in immune competence (Section 1.4.3). Macrophages are one component of a network of defense cells of diverse origin that can ingest invading microbes and foreign particles and form the reticuloendothelial system (RES). Neutrophils, eosinophils and basophils, known collectively as granulocytes or polymorphonuclear leukocytes, are important mediators of inflammatory reactions (Section 4.8). Cells of the immune system can be distinguished from one another by the expression of lineage- and maturation-specific differentiation antigens called cluster of differentiation (CD) antigens (*Table 1.3*). The CD antigens are mostly cell-surface glycoproteins that were originally defined by identifying clusters of antibodies with similar cell- and tissue-binding properties.

Table 1.1: Functions of different hematopoietic cell lineages

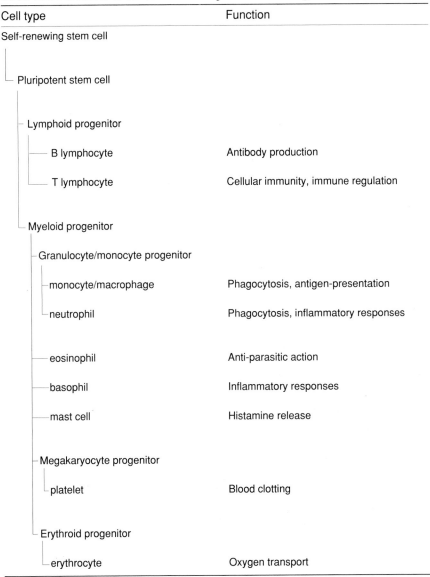

Cell type	Function
Self-renewing stem cell	
Pluripotent stem cell	
Lymphoid progenitor	
B lymphocyte	Antibody production
T lymphocyte	Cellular immunity, immune regulation
Myeloid progenitor	
Granulocyte/monocyte progenitor	
monocyte/macrophage	Phagocytosis, antigen-presentation
neutrophil	Phagocytosis, inflammatory responses
eosinophil	Anti-parasitic action
basophil	Inflammatory responses
mast cell	Histamine release
Megakaryocyte progenitor	
platelet	Blood clotting
Erythroid progenitor	
erythrocyte	Oxygen transport

Lymphocytes differentiate within the primary, or central, lymphoid organs – B cells in the bone marrow and T cells in the thymus – and then migrate into secondary, or peripheral, lymphoid organs, such as the spleen, lymph nodes and gut-associated lymphoid tissue. Lymphocytes continually circulate throughout the body in the blood, enter tissues by passing between the endothelial cells of post-capillary venules, migrate through the tissues, pass into the lymphatic circulation and then return to the blood via draining lymph nodes. The tissue distribution of lym-

Table 1.2: Cytokines involved in growth and differentiation of immune cells

Cytokine	Target cell	Principal action
Interleukin-3 (IL-3)	Myeloid progenitor	Growth and differentiation of multiple cell lineages
Granulocyte/ macrophage-CSF	Myeloid progenitor	Growth and differentiation of multiple cell lineages
(GM-CSF)	Granulocyte/monocyte progenitor	Differentiation to granulocytes and monocytes/macrophages
Granulocyte-CSF (G-CSF)	Granulocyte/monocyte progenitor	Differentiation to granulocytes
Macrophage-CSF (M-CSF)	Granulocyte/monocyte progenitor	Differentiation to monocytes/ macrophages
Interleukin-7 (IL-7)	Lymphoid progenitor	Growth and differentiation of B lymphocytes

Table 1.3: Cell surface antigens associated with lymphoid and myeloid cells

Cell type	Antigens
B lymphocyte	Surface Ig, CD19, CD20, CD21, CD22, CD23, CD37, CD38
T lymphocyte	T-cell receptor (TCR), CD2, CD3, CD4, CD5, CD7, CD8
Monocyte/macrophage	CD11b, CD11c, CD13, CD14, CD33

phocytes is determined by the binding of homing receptors present on their surface to organ-specific molecules expressed by high endothelial venules in the tissues. Cells that encounter antigen in the peripheral lymphoid tissue become activated. Activated B cells lodged within the germinal centers of lymphoid tissue are induced to proliferate and differentiate into plasma cells, the end-stage antibody-secreting cell type. Plasma cells occur in lymph nodes and spleen and also migrate to the bone marrow.

1.4.2 B lymphocytes

The essential characteristics of the antibody response to immunization (Section 1.2.3) can be explained by the selective proliferation of antigen-specific B-lymphocyte clones upon activation (*Figure 1.6*). B lymphocytes develop in the absence of any specific antigenic stimulation during the process of differentiation. Variation introduced by natural genetic mechanisms generates multiple clones of B cells (Section 1.5). Each clone contains identical B cells that express a single type of surface Ig molecule with unique V region structure and antigen-binding specificity (Section 1.3.3). B cells from different clones have distinct V region

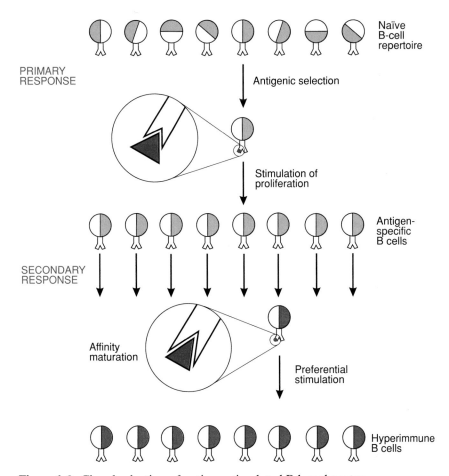

Figure 1.6: Clonal selection of antigen-stimulated B lymphocytes.

structures and hence different antigen-binding specificities. The extensive repertoire of B lymphocytes that develops in an animal is sufficiently diverse to recognize and respond to practically any foreign
antigen and to multiple epitopes on a single antigenic molecule. B cells
that recognize and bind a particular antigen proliferate selectively when
stimulated by its presence. Clonal proliferation leads to an expansion in
the number of B cells that react with the antigen. The increase in the
number of antigen-specific B cells enables the response to subsequent
immune stimulation with the same antigen to be significantly amplified.
The affinity of antigen-binding typically increases following primary
antigenic stimulation and is significantly higher in secondary responses.
The phenomenon is described as affinity maturation and is determined
by genetic mechanisms active during B-cell proliferation (Section 1.5.5).

 B lymphocytes pass through a number of stages in the course of
development from a stem cell to a mature antibody-secreting cell

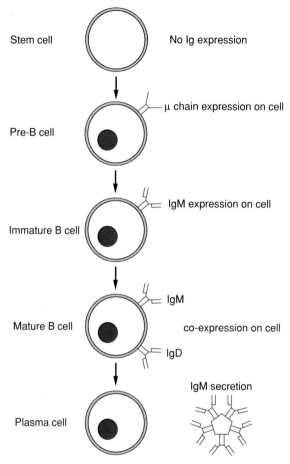

Figure 1.7: Development of B lymphocytes.

(*Figure 1.7*). Pre-B cells in the bone marrow express only μ chains. Immature B cells recently derived from bone marrow express L chains in association with μ chains and display surface IgM, although they are unresponsive to antigen at this stage. In the circulation and lymphoid tissues, mature B cells express a single type of L chain in combination with both μ and δ chains and simultaneously display surface IgM and IgD molecules with identical antigen-binding specificities. A mature B cell that binds antigen via its surface Ig becomes stimulated to prolifer- ate into a clone of identical cells. Activated B cells differentiate to pro- duce an increasing amount of secreted rather than membrane-bound IgM. The antibody-secreting plasma cell represents the final stage of B- cell maturation. The different stages of B-cell maturation are character- ized by distinct patterns of surface antigen expression (*Table 1.4*). A proportion of antigen-stimulated B cells are converted into memory B cells that survive for long periods of time and can respond to subsequent

Table 1.4: Expression of differentiation antigens during B-cell maturation

Cell type	CD19	MHC II	CD20	CD21	CD22	CD23	CD38
B-cell progenitor	+	−	−	−	−	−	+
Pre-B cell	+	+	+	−	−	−	+
Immature B cell	+	+	+	+	−	−	−
Mature B cell	+	+	+	+	+	+	−
Plasma cell	−	−	−	−	−	−	+

challenge with low levels of the specific antigen. The dominant class of Ig secreted in the primary antibody response is IgM whereas other Ig classes are predominantly secreted in secondary responses. Isotype, or class, switching occurs as the result of Ig gene rearrangement during B-cell maturation (Section 1.5.3).

1.4.3 T lymphocytes

T lymphocytes play a key role in selectively recognizing immunogens and in activating antigen-specific B lymphocytes. However, T cells do not recognize protein antigens in their native form as do B cells. Instead, T cells recognize peptide fragments of the polypeptide backbone in conjunction with specialized peptide-binding molecules of the major histocompatibility complex (MHC). The majority of cells in the body, including cells of the immune system, express MHC class I molecules. When infected with viruses, or other pathogens that replicate intracellularly, foreign proteins synthesized within a host cell are processed into peptide fragments that associate noncovalently with MHC class I molecules and are then displayed on the cell surface (*Figure 1.8*). MHC class II molecules are found on specialized antigen-presenting cells (APCs) such as macrophages, dendritic cells, B lymphocytes themselves and certain endothelial cells. APCs possess the ability to internalize extracellular antigen, process it into peptide fragments, and display the fragments on the cell surface attached noncovalently to MHC class II molecules. In humans, the class I and class II MHC genes occur in several families that are highly polymorphic. The expression of a particular combination of MHC alleles determines how an individual responds to a particular immunogen because MHC molecules differ in their structural requirements for peptide binding and so combine with different peptide fragments of the same protein antigen. The ability of T cells to recognize polymorphic differences in MHC molecules associated with the tissues of unrelated individuals underlies the phenomenon of transplant rejection (Section 4.8.5).

The cell-surface molecule of the T lymphocyte that is responsible for the specific recognition of MHC:peptide complexes is known as the

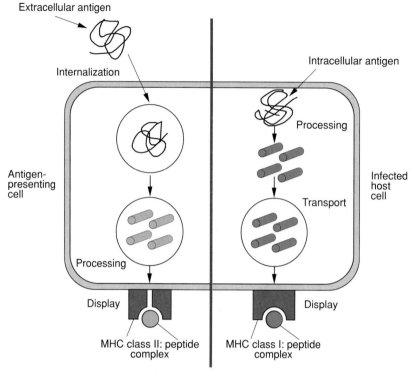

Figure 1.8: Processing and display of peptide antigens.

T-cell receptor (TCR). The TCR present on the majority of T cells is a heterodimer of α and β chains joined covalently in disulfide linkage. The α and β chains each consist of two Ig-like domains, a V domain and a C domain, with a structure that resembles the Fab portion of an antibody molecule. The Ig-like domains are linked to a transmembrane anchor and a short cytoplasmic tail. The TCRs of different T-lymphocyte clones have unique peptide-antigen-binding sites, determined by the structure of their V domains, as well as conserved regions that recognize the polymorphic determinants of the MHC molecule. The genetic mechanism by which T cells with different V domain structures arise is fundamentally similar to that involved in the generation of different antibody V domain structures (Section 1.5).

T lymphocytes are characterized by the ability to interact with cells expressing either class I or class II MHC molecules (*Figure 1.9*). Cytotoxic T lymphocytes (CTLs), or killer T cells, bear a cell-surface molecule called CD8 that binds to nonpolymorphic determinants of MHC class I molecules. Specific recognition of an MHC class I: peptide complex on a target cell by a CTL induces release of cytotoxic mediators from secretory granules that induce the death of the target cell

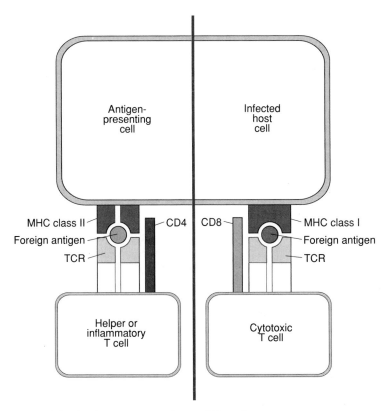

Figure 1.9: Antigen presentation to T lymphocytes.

directly. Activated CTLs also release cytokines, such as interferon-γ (IFN-γ) and tumor necrosis factor-α (TNF-α), that can up-regulate MHC class I expression and activate other cellular effector mechanisms (Section 1.6.2). T cells carrying the CD4 cell-surface molecule that binds to nonpolymorphic determinants on MHC class II molecules are of two types. Inflammatory T cells, or T_H1 cells, release IL-2, IFN-γ and TNF-β and activate macrophages that have ingested pathogens to kill the invader. Helper T cells, or T_H2 cells, release IL-4, IL-5, IL-6 and IL-10 and stimulate antigen-specific B lymphocytes to mature into antibody-secreting plasma cells (Section 1.4.4). The differentiation of CD4 +ve T cells into either T_H1 or T_H2 cells determines whether a predominantly cellular or humoral immune response to antigen is stimulated and maintained.

The TCR is stably associated with a group of membrane-associated proteins known collectively as the CD3 antigen. The interaction of an MHC:peptide complex with the TCR stimulates cytoplasmic tyrosine kinases associated with CD3, and with the CD4 or CD8 co-receptor, and triggers cell activation. The activation of antigen-specific T cells requires further signals delivered by the interaction of co-stimulatory molecules present on the surface of APCs with T-cell-surface receptors. Accessory cell-surface molecules provide additional adhesive interactions between T cells and APCs (Section 4.8). Activated T cells synthesize and secrete IL-2 and display a high-affinity receptor for the interleukin. The IL-2 receptor consists of three polypeptide chains, the α, β and γ chains. On resting T cells, only the β and γ chains are expressed to form a receptor with low affinity for IL-2. In activated T cells, the synthesis of the α chain is induced and a heterotrimeric receptor with high affinity for IL-2 is formed. IL-2 stimulation leads to the clonal proliferation of the activated T-cell clone.

1.4.4 B- and T-cell interaction

CD4 +ve, CD8 -ve helper T cells that have been appropriately activated can transduce stimulatory signals to B cells by direct cell-to-cell contact (*Figure 1.10*). B cells are themselves efficient APCs because they can bind the target antigen by means of surface Ig, internalize and process

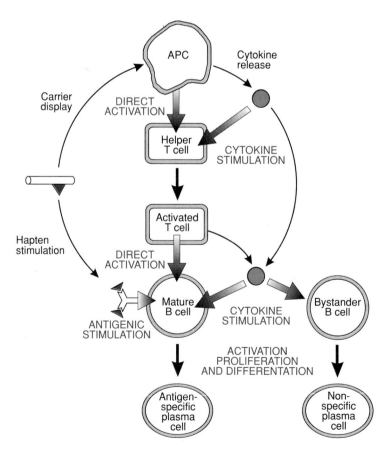

Figure 1.10: Activation of B lymphocytes during antigenic stimulation.

the antigen, and display peptide fragments of the antigen on the cell surface in association with MHC class II molecules. Accessory molecules present on the surface of the B cell provide additional adhesive interactions with T cells. Helper T cells also secrete cytokines that induce B-cell proliferation, Ig synthesis and secretion, class switching or the generation of memory B cells (Section 1.4.2). Cytokines stimulate the antigen-specific B cells that are in closest proximity to the helper T-cells. Bystander B cells can also be stimulated so that the levels of nonspecific Ig, as well as of antigen-specific Ig, become elevated. APCs also secrete cytokines that are able to promote the proliferation of both T and B lymphocytes.

The co-operation between B and T lymphocytes explains the stringent requirement for the hapten and carrier components of an immunogen to be physically linked (Section 1.2.1). The B cell recognizes the native hapten in the hapten–carrier conjugate, whereas the helper T cell recognizes peptide fragments of the carrier protein presented by the surface MHC class II molecules of APCs (*Figure 1.10*). The MHC-bound antigenic peptide fragments recognized by the TCRs of helper T cells generally differ from the protein antigenic determinants recognized by the surface Ig of B cells. Proteins and peptides are usually weakly immunogenic, or not immunogenic at all, when administered on their own. Immunogenicity can be enhanced by the co-administration of an adjuvant, a substance that enhances the process of antigen presentation and T cell stimulation. Nonpeptide antigens, such as polysaccharides and lipids, can induce antibody responses but fail to stimulate T-cell-dependent responses because they are not immunogens able to be presented to T cells by MHC molecules. The resulting T-cell-independent responses consist largely of low-affinity antibodies of the IgM class.

1.4.5 Immunological tolerance

Immunological tolerance describes the phenomenon that the immune system, which is capable of generating both T cells and antibodies recognizing practically any antigen, is restrained from reacting with the body's self antigens (Section 1.2.3). In central tolerance, immature T lymphocytes that are capable of recognizing peptide fragments of self antigens in association with MHC molecules are eliminated by programed cell death, or apoptosis. Similarly during maturation in the thymus, immature B lymphocytes are subject to clonal deletion when they encounter self antigen in the central lymphoid organs. Mature lymphocytes having the capacity to react with self antigens that are only expressed in peripheral organs or tissues, and are not present at significant levels in the central lymphoid organs during development, are not eliminated and emerge into the periphery. The binding of self antigen to peripheral T lymphocytes in the absence of the co-stimulatory signals that are provided by APCs induces a state of cellular unresponsiveness, or anergy. Similarly, mature B lymphocytes may be rendered unresponsive by interaction with self antigen in the absence of co-stimulatory signals from T cells. In peripheral tolerance, anergized lymphocytes are unable to respond to subsequent antigenic stimulation, even in combination with the normally effective co-stimulatory signals.

1.4.6 Anti-idiotypic networks

An individual can mount an antibody response against the idiotypic determinants of a foreign antibody (Section 1.3.7). Similarly, an individual can produce antibodies reactive with the idiotopes of self Ig molecules because private idiotypes have unique three-dimensional structures. Anti-idiotypic antibodies may, in turn, carry unique idiotopes that trigger further responses. The unique idiotypic structures that are presented by the membrane Ig of B cells and by the TCR of T cells can be recognized by other B- and T-cell subsets of the immune system leading to networks of cellular antibody interactions. Idiotypic networks are believed to modulate antigen-specific responses. However, the precise mechanisms involved and their importance are uncertain because the interactions are multiple and complex. Moreover, some idiotopes are located outside antigen-combining sites and are therefore common to molecules with different antigen-binding specificities.

1.5 The genetic basis of the antibody response

1.5.1 Ig genes

The organization of Ig genes is similar in humans and other mammalian species. The genes for the H chains and for the κ and λ L chains are located on different chromosomes. Ig domains and other regions of antibody structure, such as hinge regions, tail-pieces and transmembrane anchors (Sections 1.3.4 and 1.3.5), are encoded by separate regions of DNA called exons (*Figure 1.11*). Each C domain is encoded by an individual C-domain exon. The C-region exons for the H chains of each isotype are present in a single copy arranged as a tandem array. The C_κ and C_λ genes are present in a single or a few copies only. In contrast, the V_L and V_H domains have a more complex genetic origin. The amino-terminal portion of the mature V_L domain, which includes HR1 and HR2, is encoded by a V_L gene. The carboxy-terminal portion of the V_L domain is encoded by a joining (J) gene that links it to the C_L domain in the mature L chain. The HR3 of the L chain is created by the joining of V_L and J_L gene segments. Similarly, the amino- and carboxy-terminal portions of the mature V_H domain are encoded by V_H and J_H genes. In addition, a part of the V_H domain is encoded by a diversity (D) gene

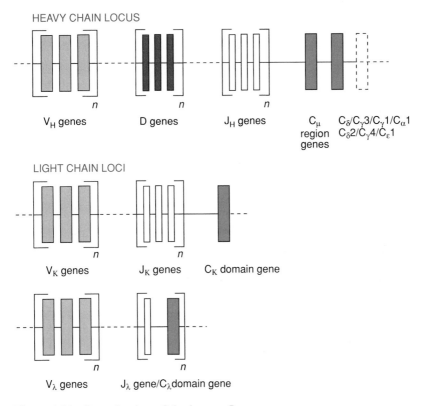

HEAVY CHAIN LOCUS

V_H genes   D genes J_H genes C_μ region genes $C_\delta/C_\gamma3/C_\gamma1/C_\alpha1$ $C_\delta2/C_\gamma4/C_\varepsilon1$

LIGHT CHAIN LOCI

V_K genes J_K genes C_K domain gene

V_λ genes J_λ gene/C_λ domain gene

Figure 1.11: Organization of the human Ig genes.

interspersed between the V_H and J_H genes. The HR1 and HR2 of the V_H domain are encoded by the V_H gene; HR3 is created by the joining of V_H, D and J_H segments. The V, D and J genes are present in multiple copies in germ line DNA. There may be up to several hundred different V genes, depending upon the species, whereas the numbers of D and J genes are more limited.

1.5.2 Ig gene rearrangement

The commitment of precursor cells to develop along the B-cell lineage is accompanied by rearrangement of germ line DNA into a functional configuration (*Figure 1.12*). Ig-gene rearrangement occurs in a series of ordered steps mediated by a system of lymphocyte-specific recombinase enzymes. The H-chain gene locus is rearranged first, with joining of a single D segment and a single J_H segment followed by joining of a single V_H gene to the D–J_H segment. The V_H–D–J_H (V_H domain) gene segment remains separated from the C-region genes by a stretch of intervening DNA. However, the rearranged V_H-domain gene segment and

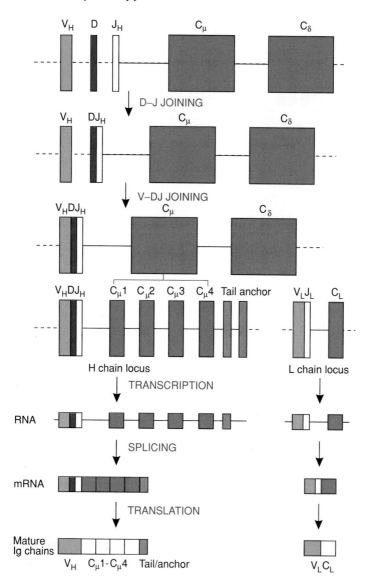

Figure 1.12: Rearrangement and expression of Ig genes.

the proximal C-region exon cluster, which encodes the μ chain, are transcribed into a single RNA molecule and the intervening sequences are spliced out to generate the mature μ-chain mRNA characteristic of the pre-B cell (Section 1.4.2). The L-chain locus becomes rearranged next, with joining of a single V_L gene to a single J_L segment. Transcription of the V_L–J_L (V_L domain) gene segment with a C_L gene and subsequent RNA splicing gives the mature L-chain mRNA. The μ and L chains associate to form the IgM that is expressed on the surface of immature B cells. Only one of the two H-chain alleles in a B lymphocyte is productively rearranged and expressed, a phenomenon termed allelic exclusion. The other H-chain allele either remains in the germ line configuration or is found to have undergone an unproductive rearrangement event. The rearrangement of L-chain genes occurs first in the κ–gene locus. Rearrangement of the λ-gene locus is precluded unless both κ alleles have first been rearranged abortively.

1.5.3 Ig-gene expression

The expression of Ig genes is controlled by lymphocyte-specific regulatory DNA sequences, such as transcriptional promoters and enhancer elements. In immature B cells, Ig chains are synthesized with leader sequences that direct their entry to the endoplasmic reticulum where the association of H and L chains and inter-chain disulfide bond formation occurs. The assembled antibody molecules are transported to the surface of the cell where they are retained in the membrane by the carboxy-terminal transmembrane anchor of the μ chain. Mature B lymphocytes express both surface IgM and surface IgD with identical V regions (Section 1.4.2). The simultaneous expression of a single V_H gene in combination with both C_μ and C_δ genes occurs by alternative splicing of a long RNA transcript that encompasses the coding sequences for both types of H chain. Following antigen stimulation, B lymphocytes begin to secrete IgM. The switch is established at the level of RNA processing: a segment coding for the transmembrane anchor and the carboxy-terminal cytoplasmic domain of the membrane form of the μ chain is replaced by one encoding the tail-piece of the secreted Ig. Class switching follows further antigenic stimulation. The mechanism of class switching involves a site-specific recombination event that deletes one or more sets of C_H exons such that the V_H-domain gene segment is juxtaposed with the next set of C_H exons along the DNA.

1.5.4 Antibody diversity

The diversity in the structure of antigen-combining sites displayed by the surface Ig of B lymphocytes in the naïve repertoire, which develops in the absence of antigenic stimulation, is determined by several factors. First, there are multiple germ line V, D and J genes capable of coming together to encode different antigen-combining sites. Second, diversity is increased by the number of different ways in which the $V_H/D/J_H$ and V_L/J_L gene segments, and the resulting V_H and V_L domains respectively, can be combined. Third, further diversity is introduced during the rearrangement of V, D and J genes. DNA rearrangement and joining is imprecise: nucleotide residues can be inserted and deleted, different reading frames of the D segments can be used, and the D segments can recombine as D–D dimers. As a result, the HR3 of the H chain is exceptionally variable in length and aa sequence. In contrast, the HR3 of the L chain, which is encoded by only two gene segments, has much more limited diversity. The potential diversity of V domain aa sequences in the primary immune repertoire is so large that it exceeds the actual number of B lymphocytes present in an individual. The true repertoire of antigen-combining specificities is probably somewhat smaller than the potential sequence repertoire because some V domains have very similar structure and some may not fold successfully to give a functional antibody molecule.

1.5.5 Affinity maturation

Affinity maturation, the increase in the affinity of antigen-specific antibodies during the course of a humoral immune response to immunization (Section 1.2.3), is the result of a genetic process that is unique to B lymphocytes. In the naïve repertoire, each B-lymphocyte clone contains a different combination of rearranged V-domain genes that encode a distinct antigen-binding specificity. Upon primary immunization, the process of antigen recognition induces proliferation of antigen-specific B lymphocytes selected from the pre-existing B-cell repertoire (Section 1.4.2). As a result, the B-cell population becomes enriched for cells with the V-domain genes that encode antigen-specific antibody. At this stage, the secreted antibody is usually of relatively low affinity. Following repeat immunization, the V-domain genes of the B cells selected after first immunization undergo somatic hypermutation. Point mutations accumulate within the V-domain genes, and the HRs in particular, during the course of repeated rounds of antigenic stimulation and cellular proliferation. Continued antigenic selection favors the proliferation of those B-cell clones with mutated V-domain genes that encode antibody of improved affinity.

1.6 Physiological properties of antibodies

1.6.1 Complement activation

Complement is a complex system of functionally-linked proteins and enzymes that are present in the blood in inactive form. The complement components are sequentially activated by a series of selective proteolytic cleavages. Triggering of the complement system at a cell surface initiates a localized cascade of enzyme activation that can result in lysis of the cell. In the classical pathway, antibody molecules that have complexed with their target antigen bind the first complement component C1. The sequential binding and activation of C1, C4 and C2 forms a complex C4b2a, that is a C3 convertase. C3 is cleaved to release a C3a fragment and a C3b fragment that binds to C4b2a to form C4b2a3b, or C5 convertase. C5 is cleaved in turn to release a C5a fragment and a C5b fragment that induces the further ordered binding of several stable complement components C6, C7, C8 and C9. C5b–C9 form a multimeric structure, called the membrane attack complex, that creates a pore in the cell membrane and leads to the death of the cell by osmotic lysis.

Antibodies of both the IgM and IgG classes can activate the complement system. Of the human IgG subclasses, IgG1 and IgG3 are most effective at activation, IgG2 is less effective and IgG4 is ineffective. The first complement protein that interacts with antibody, the multivalent C1q subcomponent, binds to monomeric IgG only weakly but binds much more strongly when several IgG molecules are aggregated in an immune complex with antigen or are arrayed on the surface of a target antigen-positive cell. C1q interacts with the $C_{\gamma}2$ domain of IgG molecules at an exposed β-strand binding motif with a characteristic aa sequence. Maximal C1q binding and complement activation depend upon the presence of the Asn-linked carbohydrate in the $C_{\gamma}2$ domain. Hinge length and flexibility of the Fab arms in the IgG molecule also influence the ability of antibody complexed with antigen to activate the complement cascade. Although IgM is a pentamer, it binds C1q only weakly until antigen binds whereupon an induced conformational change reveals further binding sites for C1q.

Antibodies that are effective triggers of complement-mediated cell lysis bind C1q and activate C1 more efficiently than poorly lytic antibodies. The efficiency of complement lysis also depends critically upon the properties of the target antigen. The density and distribution of the antigen on the target cell surface determine whether antibody Fc regions are juxtaposed in the optimal configuration for complement activation. Antibodies that bind to different epitopes on the same antigen can exhibit strongly synergistic lysis. On the other hand, some antigens are poor targets for inducing lysis because they are subject to the phenomenon of antigenic modulation. In antigenic modulation, the cross-linking of cell surface antigen molecules by bivalent or multivalent antibody results in removal of antigen and complexed antibody from the cell surface by a rapid process of internalization.

1.6.2 *Activation of cellular effector mechanisms*

Cellular effector mechanisms are triggered when IgG molecules recognize and coat the surface of foreign cells. Leukocytes employ two main mechanisms to kill antibody-coated target cells. The first mechanism is phagocytosis, a process that involves the complete engulfment of the foreign cell and its destruction by phagocytic cells such as macrophages and neutrophils. The coating of target cells with antibody to make them more attractive to phagocytic cells is called opsonization. The second mechanism, called antibody-dependent cellular cytotoxicity (ADCC),

Table 1.5: Fcγ receptors on human immune effector cells

Receptor type	Cellular distribution
FcγRI (CD64)	Macrophages Monocytes Activated neutrophils
FcγRII (CD32)	Monocytes Macrophages Neutrophils Eosinophils Platelets
FcγRIII (CD16)	NK cells Macrophages Activated monocytes Neutrophils

involves the binding and activation of large granular lymphocytes, or natural killer (NK) cells, a type of non-B non-T lymphoid cell. Activation of NK cells triggers the release of granule contents including a membrane pore-forming protein that causes osmotic lysis, a cytotoxin that activates DNA-degrading enzymes within the target cell, and various proteolytic enzymes.

The action of cellular immune mechanisms is directed by the interaction of the Fc region of antibody molecules coating the target cell with specific Fc receptors on the surface of the effector cell that transduce activation signals when cross-linked (*Table 1.5*). The high-affinity Fcγ receptor, FcγRI (CD64), displays appreciable affinity for monomeric human IgG1 and IgG3, whereas IgG4 binds with 10-fold lower affinity and IgG2 not at all. The binding site for FcγRI is in the lower hinge region of the antibody between the hinge disulfides and the amino-terminal end of the folded structure of the $C_\gamma2$ domain. The Asn-linked carbohydrate of the $C_\gamma2$ domain and the $C_\gamma3$ domain are both essential for high-affinity binding to the receptor. The interaction of target-bound antibody with immune effector cells is also influenced by hinge-region flexibility. A second receptor present on phagocytic cells, FcγRII (CD32), can bind complexed IgG, especially human IgG1 and IgG3, via a site on the antibody that probably overlaps the binding site for FcγRI. The FcγRIII (CD16) receptor binds polymeric IgG1 and IgG3 but has low affinity for monomeric IgG.

The adherence of a phagocytic cell to a target cell is promoted by complement activation. The noncatalytic complement fragment C3b deposited on the surface of the target cell can act as an opsonin by binding to complement receptors expressed by macrophages and neutrophils and thereby activating them. Other noncatalytic fragments that result from the activation of the complement cascade, C3a, C4a and C5a, stimulate immune effector cells by interacting with receptors present on a

Table 1.6: Cytokines involved in the activation of immune effector cells

Cytokine	Producer cell	Principal action
Interferon-γ (IFN-γ)	T cells (T$_H$1, CTL)	Activation of macrophages and NK cells
Tumor necrosis factor-β (TNF-β)	T cells (T$_H$1, CTL)	Activation of macrophages and neutrophils
GM-CSF	T cells (T$_H$1, CTL) Activated macrophages	Activation of monocytes and macrophages
Tumor necrosis factor-α (TNF-α)	T cells (T$_H$1, CTL) Activated macrophages	Activation of macrophages
G-CSF	Activated macrophages	Activation of neutrophils

variety of leukocytes and other cell types. C5a acts as both a chemoattractant and an activator of neutrophils. Immune effector cells are also
stimulated by cytokines that are released by cells involved in active
immune responses (*Table 1.6*).

1.6.3 Antibody distribution and metabolism

IgG is distributed throughout the body in equilibrium between the intravascular compartment and the extravascular tissues. The ability of antibody molecules to gain access to normal tissues is highly dependent
upon the anatomy of the tissue and its vascular supply. In the case of
hematopoietic and lymphoid organs, the organ-specific cells are rarely
bound to each other tightly and antibody can have relatively free access.
In bone and cartilage, on the other hand, the extracellular matrix is
dense and the convection and diffusion of macromolecules is severely
restricted. Liver, spleen and bone marrow demonstrate little resistance
to antibody infiltration of the extravascular space because the endothelium of these organs is discontinuous and the basement membrane is
absent. In contrast, the endothelium of skin and lung is much less
permeable. Connections between cells of epithelia and of organ
parenchyma, such as desmosomes and tight junctions, restrict the passage of large soluble molecules. In the brain, the vascular wall forms a
blood–brain barrier that effectively excludes both small molecules and
antibodies. The biodistribution of antibody may be altered in pathological conditions where the integrity of normal vascular barriers is compro-
mised by disease.

IgG molecules persist in the circulation of humans with the longest
half-lives of any of the serum proteins. Human IgG1, IgG2 and IgG4
have half-lives of about 3 weeks. The human IgG3 subclass has a relatively short half-life of about 1 week because of the unusually long hinge
region. The C$_\gamma$2 domain is believed to regulate the metabolic breakdown, or catabolism, of IgG independently of its ability to bind to C1q

or FcγRI. The carbohydrate residues of the $C_\gamma2$ domain contribute, in part, to the long half-life of IgG either by protecting the antibody against proteolytic digestion or by keeping the $C_\gamma2$ domains in the native conformation. However, the mechanisms by which IgG is maintained in the circulation and the sites in the body that regulate antibody catabolism remain incompletely defined. The circulating half-lives of human IgM and the other antibody classes are shorter than those of the IgG subclasses. IgM has a predominantly intravascular pattern of distribution because its larger size compared with IgG greatly restricts the ease with which it can pass out of the vascular compartment, or extravasate, and enter the tissues. The biodistribution of IgA is determined by the existence of the transepithelial transport system that conducts antibody through the interior of the epithelial cell to the mucosal surface.

1.7 Therapeutic antibodies

1.7.1 Polyclonal and monoclonal antibodies

Antiserum contains a mixture of polyclonal antibodies with multiple antigenic specificities, which are derived from multiple immune-stimulated B lymphocytes (Section 1.4.2), because the mammalian immune system has evolved to combat complex microbial pathogens and their natural variants. Polyclonal Ig comprises a mixture of antibody isotypes with greater or lesser capacity to engage the different effector elements of the immune system depending upon the target and its antigenic characteristics. The polyclonal Ig preparations obtained from immunized animals contain a relatively small proportion of antigen-specific antibodies and a larger and variable proportion of antibodies that are potentially cross-reactive with nontarget antigens and may therefore give rise to undesirable side-effects (Section 2.2). In contrast, monoclonal antibodies (Mabs), so-called because they are derived from a single clone of antibody-expressing B cells, have identical structure, antigen-binding specificity and capacity to trigger effector functions. The methodology for reliably generating Mabs to target antigen, known as hybridoma technology, was first established in rodent species (Section 2.3).

1.7.2 Animal and human antibodies

Antibodies derived from animals elicit a humoral immune response in humans (Section 1.3.7). The human antibody response leads to the formation of immune complexes with the xenogeneic Ig in the circulation and complement activation. The side-effects of immune complex formation with administered antibody, known as serum sickness, include fever, rash, joint pain and edema. Serum sickness resolves completely when all the xenogeneic antibody has been cleared by the RES. Immune complexes that persist in the circulation deposit in the basement membrane of small blood vessels where they can activate complement, trigger inflammation and cause tissue damage (Section 4.8.1). Although the side-effects are usually mild, the administration of foreign antibody risks triggering anaphylactic shock in previously sensitized individuals (Section 4.8.7). The problem of inducing antibody responses with animal Ig can be largely circumvented by the use of human polyclonal Ig preparations (Section 2.2) or human Mabs (Sections 2.3.4 and 2.3.5). However, in patients with rheumatoid arthritis (Section 4.8.4) and in some healthy individuals, there are pre-existing IgM antibodies, known as rheumatoid factors, that cross-react with antigenic determinants in the Fc regions of both human and mouse IgGs.

1.7.3 Natural and engineered antibodies

Human Mabs have proven difficult to generate routinely from immune-stimulated human B lymphocytes by means of hybridoma technology or other methodologies (Section 2.3.4). Genetic engineering techniques can be used to produce recombinant human Mabs by isolating Ig genes from human B lymphocytes and transferring them into appropriate cellular expression systems (Section 2.4.1). An alternative approach uses recombinant DNA methodology to transform well-characterized antigen-specific rodent Mabs into more human-like versions that retain the antigen-binding characteristics of the parent Mabs (Sections 2.4.2 and 2.4.3). Novel procedures that screen repertoires of V-domain genes for their antigen-binding capacity allow the isolation of human Mabs recognizing specified target antigens without the need for immunization of humans or animals (Section 2.8). Intact Ig molecules may not be ideal therapeutic agents in some clinical situations because of their relatively large size and long serum half-life. Proteolytic or recombinant fragments of antibody molecules have potential advantages as alternative therapeutic agents (Section 2.5). The therapeutic potency of Mabs can be enhanced by chemical or genetic combination with other Ig molecules and with non-Ig agents that have biological activity (Sections 2.6 and 2.7).

Chapter 2

Molecular engineering of antibodies

2.1 Introduction

The ability to tailor the structure of antibody molecules for the treatment of human disease according to the molecular target and the nature of the disorder has developed in concert with advances in several areas of technology. Hybridoma technology provides a general procedure for generating unlimited amounts of defined antigen-specific monoclonal antibodies (Mabs) from immunized rodents. Recombinant DNA manipulation may be used to engineer the structure of antibody molecules and optimize their characteristics for therapy. Genetic engineering can convert rodent Mabs into more human-like equivalents with chosen effector functions and so overcome technical limitations inherent to procedures for generating human Mabs. Antibody functions that reside within discrete folded structural elements of the Ig molecule can be isolated and manipulated independently. Structural regions involved with antigen-binding and effector functions can be separated by fragmentation of whole Ig molecules and independent Ig domains can be expressed from cloned Ig genes. Antibodies, their fragments, and recombinant analogs can be reconfigured by either chemical or genetic means and can further be combined with non-Ig entities to enhance their effectiveness. Finally, human Mabs can now be derived by *ex vivo* procedures that have the potential to bypass the need for immunization of animals and hybridoma technology altogether.

2.2 Polyclonal Ig

The immunization of domesticated animals such as horses, cows, goats, sheep and rabbits with disabled pathogens, their toxic products, or other noxious substances generates hyperimmune antisera that are enriched in antibodies specific for the immunogen. Polyclonal IgG antibody can be obtained by pooling the sera of animals, concentrating the Ig fraction, and formulating the preparation for administration (Section 5.2.1).

Human serum can be used as a source of polyclonal Ig for the prophylaxis or therapy of disease. Ig preparations from healthy human donors contain antibodies with a range of target specificities characteristic of common human pathogens as well as anti-idiotypic antibodies that may be involved in immune regulation (Section 1.4.6). However, standard Ig preparations often contain only low levels of antibody protective against a specific infectious agent. Hyperimmune human antisera can be obtained either from individuals who have already been exposed to an infection or from healthy volunteers who have consented to intentional vaccination. The sera of multiple human donors are generally pooled to isolate adequate amounts of Ig for treatment.

A source of Ig that is particularly suited to oral administration is bovine colostrum, the early milk that cows produce after giving birth, which is rich in naturally protective IgA antibodies and can be further enriched for antigen-specific antibody by immunization. The yolks of eggs laid by immunized hens are enriched for antigen-specific IgY, the avian equivalent of mammalian IgG. IgY, like human IgA, is relatively resistant to proteolytic degradation and so eggs may represent a convenient source of orally protective antibodies.

2.3 Monoclonal antibodies

B lymphocytes and antibody-secreting plasma cells generally lack the capacity to proliferate *ex vivo* and so die out after a short time in culture. The ability to produce Mabs relies upon a method that can stably preserve the functional capacity of B cells and allow the sorting and identification of clones of cells that express particular antigen-specific Mabs. Immune B lymphocytes can be fused with myeloma cell lines to create hybrid cell lines, or hybridomas, that are able to reproduce in culture and secrete antibody continuously. Myelomas are tumors of the B-cell lineage that are characterized by rapid proliferation and the secretion of large quantities of abnormal Igs called myeloma proteins. Myeloma cell lines that have lost the capacity to synthesize their own Ig chains are the favored fusion partners for B lymphocytes. The Mabs secreted by hybridomas derived from such myeloma lines consist of the single H and L chains originally expressed by the parent B cell and are unispecific and bivalent like the parent antibody.

2.3.1 Rodent Mabs

Mabs are most commonly raised following immunization of mice. Mouse spleen cells are fused with mouse myeloma cell lines that can multiply indefinitely in long-term culture to create mouse hybridomas (*Figure 2.1*). The hybridoma cell inherits the capacity of the myeloma cell for continuous proliferation and the capacity of the spleen B cell to synthesize and secrete Ig. Typically, splenic immune lymphocytes are mixed with myeloma cells under conditions that promote cell–cell

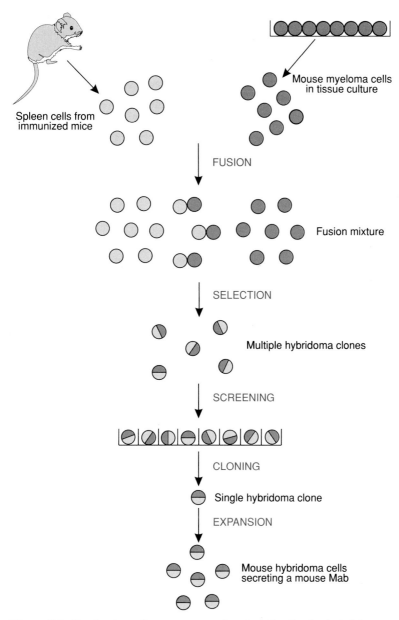

Figure 2.1: Production of mouse monoclonal antibodies by hybridoma technology.

fusion. The cell mixture is then transferred to a selection medium that favors the outgrowth of the hybridoma cells. Hybridomas secreting mouse Mab with the desired antigen-recognition characteristics of target specificity and high avidity are identified by means of screening assays, are subcloned to ensure monoclonality, and are then expanded in number. Rat Mabs can also be obtained routinely by immunization and the application of similar hybridoma technology.

Hybridoma cell lines may be grown in mice and the secreted Mab harvested either from the peritoneum or from blood. In this case, the Mab preparation is contaminated with normal mouse Ig of irrelevant antigen-binding specificity. Alternatively, hybridoma lines can be grown in continuous tissue culture systems to generate Mab that is not contaminated by Ig molecules with irrelevant antigen-binding properties. Cell culture allows the reproducible manufacture of antigen-specific Mab in bulk by large-scale fermentation procedures (Section 5.2.2).

2.3.2 Properties of mouse and rat Mabs

In the mouse, the IgG subclasses are denoted IgG1, IgG2a, IgG2b and IgG3. In the rat, the IgG subclasses are denoted IgG1, IgG2a, IgG2b and IgG2c. The IgG subclasses within and across human and rodent species differ in their aa sequences, in the number and pattern of inter-chain disulfide bonds and in their physiological properties. The mouse subclasses IgG2a, IgG2b and IgG3 and the rat isotypes IgG1, IgG2a and IgG2b are able to activate complement. Mouse IgG2a and rat IgG2b antibodies contain the binding site aa sequence that is present in all the IgG isotypes that bind to the human FcγRI receptor (Section 1.6.2) and are able to trigger phagocytosis by human effector cells. Mouse and rat Mabs have considerably shorter half-lives in humans than endogenous human IgG despite the similarities in Ig structure.

Mouse Mabs administered to humans elicit a humoral immune response that is commonly referred to as a human anti-mouse antibody (HAMA) response. Although mouse Mabs invoke a response that is predominantly directed against the species-specific isotypic determinants, a significant component of the HAMA response is also directed against the idiotypic determinants (Section 1.3.7). The development of the HAMA response can markedly accelerate the clearance of mouse antibody from the circulation, interfere with its ability to extravasate and block its capacity to bind to target antigen in the tissues. Similarly, rat antibodies stimulate a human anti-rat antibody response.

2.3.3 Univalent and bispecific Mabs

The capacity of hybridomas to synthesize and assemble Ig chains and to secrete intact Mab can be exploited to produce variant Mabs with a single functional antigen-combining site or with two sites recognizing different target antigens. The fusion of a B lymphocyte with a myeloma cell line that secretes L chain of irrelevant antigen-binding specificity

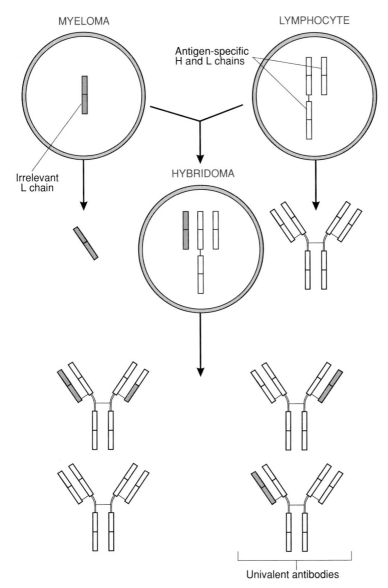

Figure 2.2: Univalent monoclonal antibodies by hybridoma technology.

creates a hybridoma line that manufactures a mixed population of antibody molecular (*Figure 2.2*). The single type of H chain expressed can associate with both the antigen-specific L chain and the irrelevant L chain. The secreted Mab consists, in major part, of univalent antibody with a single functional antigen-combining site. The univalent Mab fraction can generally be purified from the two bivalent Mab forms in reasonable overall yield. Bispecific Mabs with dual antigen-combining specificity can be produced by fusing two hybridoma cell lines, each of

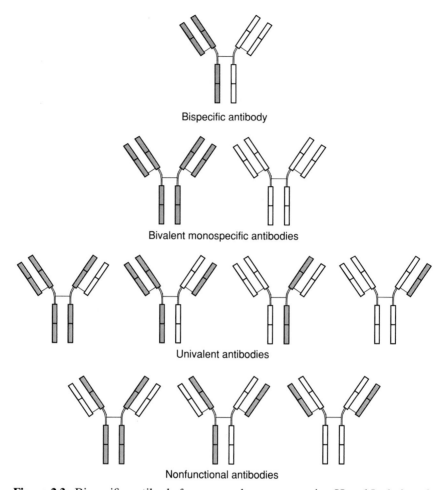

Bispecific antibody

Bivalent monospecific antibodies

Univalent antibodies

Nonfunctional antibodies

Figure 2.3: Bispecific antibody from a quadroma expressing H and L chains of two Ig molecules.

which secretes a single type of Mab with unique antigen-binding specificity. The resultant hybrid hybridomas, also known as quadromas, synthesize the H and L chains derived from both parental hybridoma lines co-dominantly. The association of H/H and H/L chains in all combinations can theoretically lead to the assembly of 10 different forms of Mab (*Figure 2.3*). Assuming that the different Ig chains are synthesized in equal amounts and associate completely at random, the bispecific Mab fraction represents one-eighth of the total synthesized Mab. The yield of bispecific Mab varies in practice because certain Ig-chain combinations occur preferentially, and purification of the bispecific from the complex mixture of other Mab types can be difficult. The pairing of two H chains of different isotype can alter or abolish the ability of the Fc region in the bispecific Mab to trigger immune effector functions.

2.3.4 Human Mabs

The generation of human antigen-specific Mabs is more problematic than the production of Mabs from immunized rodents. Activated B lymphocytes can be obtained from patients who have mounted an active immune response to antigens characteristic of microbial disease, cancer or autoimmune disease (Chapter 4). However, humans cannot generally be immunized to obtain therapeutic Mabs that have human antigen-binding specificity on practical as well as ethical grounds. Methods that allow the immune stimulation of naïve human B lymphocytes with antigen *ex vivo*, can potentially circumvent this limitation. However, *in vitro* immunization tends to induce primary immune responses that involve IgM antibodies of low to intermediate affinity and limited diversity. Whether obtained by immunization *in vitro* or *in vivo*, the resultant immune B cells must be immortalized to be turned into useful antibody-producing lines.

The conventional hybridoma methodology is technically more demanding to apply to the production of human Mabs than of rodent Mabs (Section 2.3.1). Human myeloma cell lines tend to grow poorly in culture and to secrete relatively low levels of Ig compared with rodent myeloma lines. The usual source of human cells for fusion, peripheral blood, contains few immune cells actively involved in the antibody response compared with the spleen or lymph nodes. A number of alternative strategies to create stable cell lines able to secrete antigen-specific human Mabs in culture have been devised.

EBV transformation. Strains of the Epstein–Barr virus (EBV) can establish a latent and essentially nonreplicative infection in B cells leading to transformation, Ig secretion and indefinite cell proliferation. Although EBV-transformed lymphoblastoid cell lines grow well in culture, they can be unstable and produce low amounts of Mab.

Mouse myeloma fusion. Human B cells can be fused with conventional mouse myeloma cell lines to generate hybridoma cells with high frequency. However, such mouse/human hybridomas tend to be unstable and to eliminate human chromosomes preferentially when maintained in culture.

Heteromyeloma fusion. Heteromyeloma lines formed by fusing a human lymphoid tumor line with a nonsecreting mouse myeloma cell line are more suitable fusion partners for human cells. The resulting heterohybridomas, or triomas, tend to be relatively stable and to secrete higher levels of human Mab.

In practice, a combination of methodologies may need to be tried to ensure the creation of a useful cell line that produces a human Mab. In the case of unstable hybridoma cell lines, the genes encoding the V domains of an antigen-specific human Mab can be rescued and cloned into stable and efficient Mab expression systems (Section 2.4).

2.3.5 Human Mabs from mice

An alternative approach to the generation of human Mabs attempts to build elements of the human immune system into the mouse. Strains of mice carrying a genetic mutation that disables the recombinase system (Section 1.5.2) suffer from severe combined immunodeficiency disease (SCID) and completely lack functional T and B lymphocytes. SCID mice can accept grafts of normal human cells without the rejection that normally accompanies transplantation of tissue from another species (Section 1.4.3). Thus, SCID mice can be repopulated with normal human lymphocytes to provide a source of immune B cells for the production of human Mabs. Although primary immunization has not proven routinely effective, human lymphocytes that have already been primed can be stimulated by antigen to produce large secondary responses following transfer to SCID mice.

Mice capable of making human Mabs directly in response to primary antigenic stimulation have been created by genetic manipulation. Human Ig genes can be introduced either into fertilized oocytes or into embryonic stem cells *ex vivo* and the cells then implanted into a surrogate mother to develop. Strains of transgenic mice with the desired characteristics are produced by breeding from the progeny. The transfer of the large DNA segments that would be required to carry all the human Ig genes into mouse cells is technically difficult. Instead, human Ig-gene miniloci, which include a limited number of V domain and C region genes for each of the H and L chains, have been constructed by the joining of noncontiguous fragments of germ line DNA and introduced into mice. The human Ig genes present in transgenic mice can be productively rearranged in a physiologically relevant manner, undergo V–(D)–J joining, H-chain class switching and somatic hypermutation to generate a repertoire of antigen-specific human antibodies (Section 1.5). An important refinement of transgenic mouse technology is the creation of strains in which the functions of the endogenous mouse H and L chain loci have been knocked out by targeted gene disruption so that animals carrying integrated human DNA make only human antibody upon immunization.

2.4 Recombinant Mabs

Hybridoma cell lines can undergo rare and spontaneous genetic mutation events that lead to Ig class or subclass switching, to deletion or replacement of C-region domains, or to alterations in antibody affinity and specificity. Such processes occur in an undirected fashion and cannot easily be used to alter antibody characteristics in a deliberate way. In functionally rearranged Ig genes, intervening DNA sequences separate the V domain and the individual C domain coding regions (Section 1.5.1). This genetic arrangement permits the directed recombination of different V-domain genes with C-region genes of different isotype or species by genetic engineering techniques.

The DNA sequences encoding the V_H and V_L domains of a Mab can be isolated by using the polymerase chain reaction (PCR) to amplify cDNA obtained from an antibody-expressing hybridoma cell. Oligonucleotide primers are designed that are complementary to the nucleotide sequences present at each end of the rearranged V-domain gene segments of the H and L chains. The primers also incorporate specific restriction enzyme sites to enable precise cloning of the amplified DNA into appropriate expression vectors (Section 2.4.1). By this method, V-domain genes can be recovered from stable hybridomas, unstable human antibody-producing cells or nonsecreting B cells, and Mabs with the natural antigen-recognition properties recovered by expression of recombinant Ig gene vectors that pair the cloned V-domain genes with genes encoding selected C domains (*Figure 2.4*).

2.4.1 Antibody expression systems

Cloned antibody genes can be expressed in a number of different cell types. Myeloma cells are the natural choice for the expression of recombinant Ig genes because they have evolved the cellular machinery to recognize Ig gene regulatory signals and so express the genes at high levels, to assemble the H and L chains and glycosylate them appropriately, and to secrete the intact antibody molecule efficiently. To express an intact recombinant Mab, the cloned H and L chain genes must both be transfected into a myeloma cell line that does not produce its own Ig chains. DNA vectors have been designed that allow propagation and selection of recombinant plasmids in *Escherichia coli*. The vectors also contain dominant selectable markers that allow isolation of transfectant myeloma cells, or transfectomas, that are capable of expressing intact Mab. The expression levels of Ig genes can be much poorer in transfectomas than in hybridoma cell lines because the expression vectors lack certain enhancer elements. High-level expression of intact antibody molecules is possible using alternative mammalian expression systems based on Chinese hamster ovary, or CHO, cells. Vectors that incorporate appropriate resistance markers allow selection of transfected cells that contain amplified copies of the vector sequence and consequently produce higher levels of Mab.

Ig chains can be expressed in *E. coli* although the reducing environment of the bacterial cell cytoplasm inhibits correct disulfide bond for-

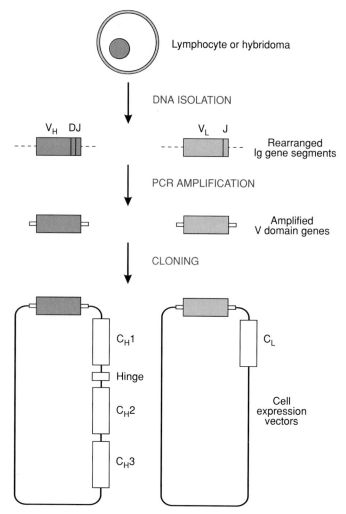

Figure 2.4: Cloning V domain genes into expression vectors.

mation and the expressed H and L chains accumulate in insoluble form within inclusion bodies. Functional antibody molecules can only be obtained by recovering the Ig chains from the inclusion bodies and renaturating them under oxidizing conditions that promote disulfide bonding. *E. coli* is also incapable of adding oligosaccharide side-chains to Ig chains, a feature known to influence the physiological properties of intact antibody molecules (Section 1.3.6). Nonmammalian eukaryotic cells derived from yeasts, insects and plants can assemble intact glycosylated antibody molecules and secrete them. However, Mabs from these expression hosts do not invariably retain natural physiological functions because the patterns of protein glycosylation in such cells differ substantially from those of mammalian cells.

Techniques have been developed that permit the stable integration of transgenes in the germ line DNA of cows, sheep and goats. In addition, vector systems have been devised to drive the synthesis and secretion of foreign proteins encoded by the transgene selectively in the lactating mammary gland. In principle, therapeutic Mabs can be isolated in bulk from the milk of transgenic animals created by the introduction of antigen-specific Ig genes.

2.4.2 Chimeric Mabs

A rodent Mab can be rendered more human-like by replacing its C domains with human equivalents by genetic manipulation (*Figure 2.5*). The most common approach is to transfer the antigen-specific V_H- and V_L-domain genes, which have been cloned from the rodent hybridoma, to expression vectors carrying the human C_H- and C_L-region genes respectively. A different strategy employs homologous recombination. The rodent hybridoma cell line is transfected with a plasmid that carries human C-region genes flanked by DNA sequences corresponding to those around the rodent C-region genes. The introduced DNA can recombine with the rodent genes, leading to insertion of the human sequences in place of the rodent DNA, although such events occur with low frequency. Rodent/human chimeric Mabs generally retain the antigen-binding specificity and affinity of the Fab arms from the rodent Mab. In some instances, a chimeric Mab does not exactly mimic the binding properties of the parent rodent Mab because the human isotype can influence the way in which the Fab arms interact with antigen. Chimeric Mabs activate effector functions according to the properties of

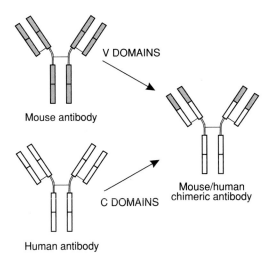

Figure 2.5: Structure of mouse–human chimeric antibody.

the human Fc region, are less immunogenic in humans than rodent Mabs, and have a significantly longer serum half-life.

'Primatized' Mabs are antibodies in which V_H and V_L domains derived from a nonhuman primate species are linked to human C regions. The FR sequences of the V domains from the cynomolgus macaque demonstrate high homology with those of human V domains. Thus, macaque/human chimeric Mabs should resemble human antibodies more closely than rodent/human chimeric Mabs. Importantly, the immune system of the macaque differs sufficiently from that of the human in that it can mount a humoral response against even the relatively conserved epitopes of human antigens.

2.4.3 Humanized Mabs

Rodent Mabs can be 'humanized' more completely by replacing the FRs of the V domains with human equivalents while retaining the CDRs of the rodent antibody that determine its antigen-binding properties (*Figure 2.6*). In practice, this straightforward approach to CDR grafting generally does not lead to reconstitution of the original affinity of antigen binding. The reason is that non-CDR aa residues also determine whether the grafted rodent CDRs are supported by human V_H and V_L frameworks in the native antigen-binding conformation, and some FR aa residues participate directly in antigen binding (Section 1.3.3). A number of strategies can be adopted to engineer humanized Mabs of acceptable antigen-binding affinity. The strategies rely upon knowledge of a large number of rodent and human V domain aa sequences, the three-dimensional crystal structures of a smaller number of Mabs or Mab fragments, and upon extensive computer modeling of antibody

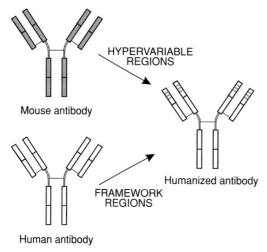

Figure 2.6: Structure of humanized mouse antibody.

structure. The dual aims of these strategies are to select the appropriate human analog of any particular rodent V_H or V_L domain as the base for CDR grafting and to introduce the minimal number of aa residue alterations into the humanized V domains to improve antigen-binding affinity.

Reshaping. The V_H and V_L domains of the rodent Mab are compared with a consensus aa sequence for the relevant family of rodent genes. This step identifies FR aa residues that may have become mutated during affinity maturation, are therefore presumed to be critical to antibody affinity and may need to be included in the humanized Mab. The human V-domain framework selected for nearest equivalence to the rodent framework is, in turn, compared with its family consensus aa sequence to highlight any residues that are idiosyncratic and may need to be substituted by consensus or equivalent germ line aa residues. Further aa residues derived from the sequence of the rodent Mab may be introduced in regions adjacent to the CDRs to approximate more closely the natural binding conformation of the rodent Mab (*Figure 2.7*).

Hyperchimerization. The V domain aa sequences of the rodent Mab are compared to the available human V domain aa sequences and the human aa sequences with the highest homology are selected as the acceptor frameworks. Idiosyncratic aa residues in the human FRs are replaced with consensus aa residues. Structural modeling is then used to identify any FR aa residues that are predicted to interact with the CDRs and so may need to be substituted to enable the CDR loops to assume the appropriate conformation for antigen binding. The procedure can generate humanized Mabs with affinities that approximate to those of the parent rodent Mabs without the need to compare alternative constructions generated by experimental reshaping.

Resurfacing. The structure of the rodent V domains is altered so that the aa residues on the exterior surface of the Mab are replaced with human equivalents selected from V domain aa sequences with the highest homology. The distribution of surface-exposed aa residues relative to the primary sequence is highly conserved between Mabs of the same species. The sequence alignment positions of surface residues in human and mouse V domains are also conserved so that only a limited number of aa residues need be substituted to convert between mouse and human. The strategy preserves the aa residues within the interior of the V domains that are critical for the proper folding of each V domain and for the packing together of the V_H and V_L domains in the correct antigen-binding conformation.

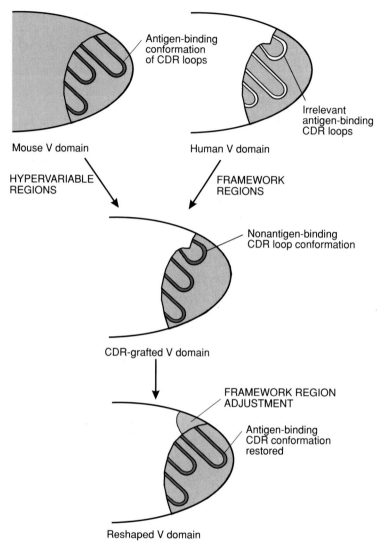

Figure 2.7: Antibody humanization by CDR-grafting and reshaping.

Compared with rodent/human chimeric Mabs, in which the rodent aa sequences comprise about 30% of the total Ig structure, humanized Mabs can have as little as 3% rodent-derived aa sequence and are therefore potentially much less immunogenic in humans. The unique idiotype of the humanized Mab may nevertheless be recognized as foreign by the human immune system. In addition, certain allotypes of human C regions may prove immunogenic or provide carrier determinants that enhance anti-idiotypic responses in individuals with different allotypic determinants. Humanized Mabs have a longer serum half-life than their rodent counterparts. However, rodent cell lines glycosylate Ig molecules slightly differently to human cells and the differences in carbohydrate structure can adversely influence the metabolism of humanized Mabs relative to endogenous human Ig.

2.5 Antibody fragments

2.5.1 Proteolytic antibody fragments

The extended hinge region of IgG molecules (Section 1.3.4) is readily accessible to proteinases, whereas the compactly folded Ig domains are relatively resistant to proteolysis. Susceptibility to proteolytic cleavage on the amino- or carboxy-terminal side of the disulfide-bonded part of the hinge depends upon the precise aa sequence and upon the presence or absence of *O*-linked oligosaccharide side-chains. Papain cleaves IgG antibodies on the amino-terminal side of the hinge to release two identical univalent Fab fragments (50 kDa approx.) and an Fc fragment (50 kDa approx.) that retains the intact disulfide-linked portion of the hinge (*Figure 2.8*). The two polypeptide chains of the Fab fragment, the L chain and a portion of the H chain called the Fd fragment, are held together by strong noncovalent interactions as well as by the covalent inter-chain disulfide bond. Pepsin cleaves IgG antibodies on the carboxy-terminal side of the hinge to release a bivalent F(ab′)$_2$ fragment (100 kDa approx.), in which the two Fab arms remain connected by the hinge disulfides, and an Fc′ fragment that usually becomes further digested into smaller peptides (*Figure 2.8*). The two Fab′ arms of the F(ab′)$_2$ fragment do not interact other than through the disulfide-bonded hinge region. Under mild reducing conditions that split disulfide bonds, F(ab′)$_2$ fragments dissociate into univalent Fab′ fragments that carry one or more Cys thiol groups, depending upon the isotype. The presence of thiol groups in Fab′ fragments generated by proteolysis is especially useful for chemical modification or conjugation (Section 2.6).

Antibody fragments can be generated from polyclonal Ig and Mabs, with known antigen-binding affinity and specificity, quickly, cheaply and in bulk by the proteolytic approach. In general, human and rodent IgGs show characteristic patterns of cleavage with papain, pepsin and other proteases according to their isotype. However, the conditions of proteolysis need to be optimized for each antibody individually, and the yields of antibody fragments can be poor if cleavage at the hinge is not favored, if competing fragmentations occur or if purification proves to be complex. Univalent antigen-binding Fab/c fragments (100 kDa approx.) and Fv fragments (25 kDa approx.) have been generated successfully by a proteolytic approach in some cases (*Figure 2.8*).

Antibody Fab, Fab′ and F(ab′)$_2$ fragments distribute from the blood into the peripheral tissues more rapidly than intact IgG because their smaller size means that they are better able to cross capillary barriers

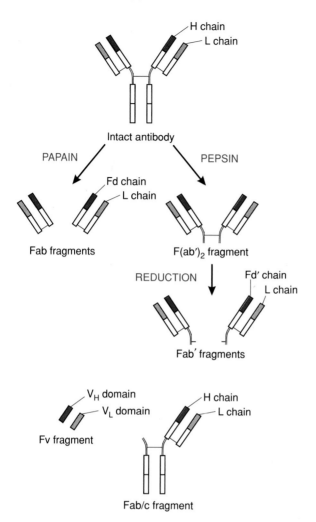

Figure 2.8: Antigen-binding proteolytic fragments of IgG.

and to diffuse across interstitial spaces (Section 1.6.3). However, antibody fragments of diminishing size become increasingly subject to glomerular filtration by the kidneys. Thus, Fab and Fab′ fragments are cleared more rapidly from the circulation than the larger $F(ab')_2$ fragments. Fc fragments and other antibody fragments that retain an intact Fc region distribute into the tissues more rapidly than intact antibody but have similar rates of catabolism to IgG.

2.5.2 Recombinant antibody fragments

Recombinant DNA technology exploits the fact that individual antibody domains are encoded by distinct Ig exons to produce Fv, Fab, Fab′, Fc and completely novel antibody molecules. A major advantage of the recombinant approach is that it can be applied, in principle, to the Ig genes of any antibody irrespective of species of origin and isotype. In common with Mabs, recombinant antibody fragments can be produced in both mammalian and eukaryotic cell systems. However, in contrast with the inability of prokaryotic expression systems to make intact antibody molecules efficiently (Section 2.4.1), bacterial expression systems have proven valuable for the production of antibody fragments. Antigen-binding Fab and Fab' fragments consist of only two heterologous polypeptide chains and are not generally glycosylated. Expression strategies have been developed by which recombinant Ig chains synthesized in the cytoplasm of the bacterium are transported to the periplasm, the space located between the cell membrane and the cell wall. The Ig chains are linked genetically to signal sequences that transport them to the periplasm and are then cleaved off to release the mature recombinant chain. In contrast with Ig gene expression in the cytoplasm (Section 2.4.1), intra- and inter-chain disulfide bonds form correctly and functional antibody fragments assemble within the oxidative environment of the periplasm.

Antibody L and Fd chains (*Figure 2.8*) can be expressed simultaneously in *E. coli*, fold independently and associate to form functional Fab fragments within the periplasm. Similarly, recombinant Fab' fragments are produced by cells expressing L chain and an Fd' chain that contains a carboxy-terminal extension corresponding to a portion of a natural antibody hinge region or an artificial aa sequence containing one or more Cys residues (Section 2.7.2). Fv fragments with antigen-binding ability can be produced by *E. coli* cells transfected with expression vectors that encode the V_H and V_L domains. The Fv fragment heterodimers are less stable than Fab or Fab' fragments because the strength of non-covalent association between the V_H and V_L domains is weaker than that between L and Fd chains, and because there is no natural disulfide bond between the two V domains. The V_H and V_L chains can be linked covalently by substituting a single aa residue at an appropriate site in each V domain with a Cys residue so that a novel disulfide linkage is created at the interface between the two chains (*Figure 2.9*). Another tactic genetically links the V_H and V_L domains by means of an oligopeptide spacer that spans the distance between the carboxy terminus of one chain and the amino terminus of the other chain in either orientation. The use of a hydrophilic and flexible peptide linker that allows the two V domains to associate without disrupting their conformation creates a single-chain Fv (scFv) fragment with antigen-binding capacity (*Figure 2.9*). The smaller size of scFv fragments allows them to distribute into tissues and to clear from the circulation more rapidly than Fab or Fab' fragments (Section 2.5.1).

Isolated H or L chains and individual recombinant V domains, also called single-domain antibodies (*Figure 2.9*), can exhibit antigen binding

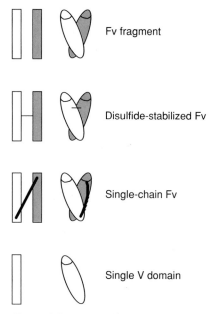

Figure 2.9: Recombinant V domain fragments.

properties similar to those of the parent Mab. V_H domains have a greater potential for diversity in HR3 and generally provide a major contribution to the interaction with antigen (Sections 1.3.2 and 1.3.3). However, V_H domains usually bind with lower affinity and specificity compared with Fab or Fab' fragments because any interactions that the antigen may make with the V_L domain are absent. The extent of interaction of the V_H domain with antigen may be enhanced by manipulating a non-CDR loop in FR3 to create the equivalent of a fourth CDR. A second disadvantage is that the hydrophobic face of the V_H domain, which normally interacts with the V_L domain, becomes exposed when the domain is isolated, and promotes aggregation. In principle, the substitution of hydrophobic aa residues at the interface surface with hydrophilic aa residues can enhance the solubility of V_H domains. Interestingly, functional IgG-like molecules found in camelid species contain H chains that lack a C_H1 domain and are devoid of L chains. The unpaired camelid V_H domains form the basis for the design of soluble single-domain antibodies.

2.5.3 Antigen-binding mimetics

Protein engineering has been used to create novel antigen-binding polypeptides based on the structure of antibodies. One such recombinant protein, called a minibody, was designed to mimic a portion of the V_H domain that includes the first and second HRs (Section 1.3.2). The protein incorporates three β-strands from each of the two β-sheets as well as the HR1 and HR2 loops. Amino acid substitutions were incorporated to make the conformations of the CDR loops similar to those in the natural V domain and to replace any hydrophobic aa residues that are not normally exposed.

Antibody CDRs have been termed 'minimal recognition units' because synthetic oligopeptides based on the aa sequence of CDR loops can demonstrate the ability to recognize antigen. However, such peptides usually bind antigen less strongly than the Mab by several orders of magnitude even when they are conformationally constrained to better mimic the three-dimensional orientation of the CDR loops in the Mab. A detailed knowledge of the structure of CDRs and their interaction with antigen, or computer predictions of CDR conformation, can form the basis for the rational design and synthesis of non-peptide mimetic compounds with the ability to bind antigen.

2.6 Antibody conjugates

2.6.1 Conjugation chemistry

Antibody molecules, in common with other proteins, contain a variety of aa residues – especially tyrosine (Tyr) and lysine (Lys) – with side-chain functional groups that can act as sites of chemical modification or covalent attachment. Antibody Fab' fragments carry a segment of the hinge region that includes one or more Cys residues with reactive thiol groups at the carboxy-terminal end of the molecule (Section 2.5.1). The location of the hinge Cys residues at a site distant from the antigen-combining site of the fragment minimizes the risk that chemical conjugation will interfere with antigen binding. Although intact IgG molecules rarely contain Cys residues that are not involved in disulfide bonding, the oligosaccharide side-chains of the $C_\gamma 2$ domains represent a useful site of modification at a location away from the antigen-combining sites (Section 1.3.6).

Tyrosine residues. The phenolic side-chain of Tyr residues is susceptible to substitution by highly reactive and relatively nonspecific electrophilic agents. Selective iodination of the Tyr side-chain is a common procedure used to introduce radioisotopes for labeling and therapy (Sections 3.6.1 and 4.2).

Lysine residues. The amino group, $-NH_2$, of the Lys side-chain can be reacted under mild conditions with a variety of reagents that leave other aa side-chains largely unmodified. Agents bearing activated carboxylic esters of general structure Y–CO–R (where Y is an activating group and R is the chemical backbone) react to give chemically stable amide bonds with the structure: *Antibody*–NH–CO–R.

Cysteine residues. The thiol group, –SH, of the Cys side-chain possesses unique chemical characteristics that allow it to be modified selectively under mild conditions. Reagents that contain a highly reactive disulfide bond, X–SS–R (where X is an activating group), form reducible disulfide bonds: *Antibody–SS–R*. Reagents that contain an alkylating group, Z–R (where Z is an alkyl halide or a maleimide group), form non-reducible thioether bonds: *Antibody–S–R*.

Oligosaccharide side-chains. Antibody-linked carbohydrate can be oxidized chemically under conditions that have little or no effect on the structure of the polypeptide. The procedure generates aldehyde groups, *Antibody–CHO*, able to react with agents that bear reactive amino groups, $R-NH_2$, to form covalent bonds that can be made stable by subsequent reduction to the secondary amine: *Antibody–CH$_2$–NH–R*.

Antibody conjugates, or immunoconjugates, that incorporate low-molecular-weight entities are commonly synthesized by using a chemical derivative of the ligand that has been activated to react with aa side-chain groups of the Ig molecule. The attachment of larger ligands is generally achieved by using chemical cross-linking agents that modify aa residues as selectively as possible so as to leave unaltered the antigen-binding characteristics and effector functions of the antibody (Section 2.6.3). Bifunctional cross-linking agents contain two chemically reactive groups linked by an inert chemical backbone. The cross-linker first attaches to antibody via one of the chemically reactive groups and, in so doing, introduces the second chemically reactive group, which is then capable of reacting with another protein or ligand molecule. Two different types of cross-linker are commonly used: homobifunctional agents contain two identical reactive groups whereas heterobifunctional agents contain two distinct chemical groups that are reactive under different conditions. Amino acid residues critical to Ig function can be unintentionally modified, especially at high substitution ratios, and so the number of ligand or cross-linker molecules that can be attached to a single antibody molecule is limited.

2.6.2 Conjugates of antibody fragments

Antibody molecules with two identical antigen-combining sites can be constructed by chemically coupling two identical univalent Fab′ fragments. Similarly, bivalent antibodies with dual antigen-binding specificity can be made by joining two Fab′ fragments derived from different antibodies. Fab′ fragments are chemically coupled by one of two approaches (*Figure 2.10*). In the simplest case, the free thiol group of a Fab′ fragment, Fab′$_A$ is modified by attachment of an activating group, Fab′$_A$–SS–X. Reaction with a second Fab′ fragment, Fab′$_B$, bearing a

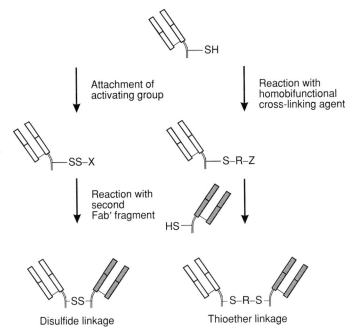

Figure 2.10: Synthesis of Fab′ dimers by chemical conjugation.

free thiol group produces a Fab′ dimer linked by a disulfide bond, Fab′$_A$–SS–Fab′$_B$. Alternatively, a Fab′ fragment is first reacted with an excess of a homobifunctional alkylating agent, Z–R–Z. This step introduces a reactive alkylating group, Fab′$_A$–S–R–Z, which can then react with the thiol group of the second Fab′ fragment to give a Fab′ dimer linked by two thioether bonds, Fab′$_A$–S–R–S–Fab′$_B$. Nonreducible thioether bonds have the potential advantage over disulfide bonds that they are resistant to splitting by reducing agents. The reduction of an exposed disulfide bond *in vivo* can lead to dissociation of the Fab′ arms. More complex conjugation procedures are required when Fab′ fragments containing several reactive thiol groups are cross-linked. Fab′ dimers with multiple inter-chain disulfide bonds are more stable to breakdown by reduction.

Multimeric Fab′ conjugates can be synthesized by the use of more complex polyfunctional cross-linkers or more elaborate conjugation procedures (Section 3.4.2). Fab′ fragments can also be endowed with antibody-like properties by chemical attachment to isolated Fc fragments. The proteolytic Fc fragment of human polyclonal IgG, which is predominantly of the IgG1 subclass, contains a hinge region with two disulfide bonds (Section 1.3.4). The thiol groups of one of these bonds can be used to attach one or more Fab′ fragments in hinge-to-hinge linkage with a single Fc fragment using homobifunctional alkylating agents, or to attach one or more Fab′ fragments to a chemically-coupled Fc dimer.

2.6.3 Antibody–protein conjugates

Antibody–protein conjugates are commonly synthesized using bifunctional cross-linking agents (Section 2.6.1). Homobifunctional cross-linking agents that react with the amino groups of Lys residues are generally unsuitable because they can cross-link protein molecules internally and produce homologous as well as heterologous conjugate molecules. Heterobifunctional cross-linking agents that exploit the chemical properties of Cys thiol groups permit more efficient conjugation in a generally applicable two-step scheme (*Figure 2.11*). The first step in the process involves reaction of the antibody and a cross-linker, Y–CO–R–SS–X, that introduces an activated disulfide bond, *Antibody*–NH–CO–R–SS–X. The second protein component may naturally contain a Cys thiol group, this may be engineered into a recombinant molecule, or it may be introduced by means of a cross-linking agent. Reaction of the derivatized antibody with *Protein*-SH in the second step creates a disulfide-linked immunoconjugate with the structure: *Antibody*

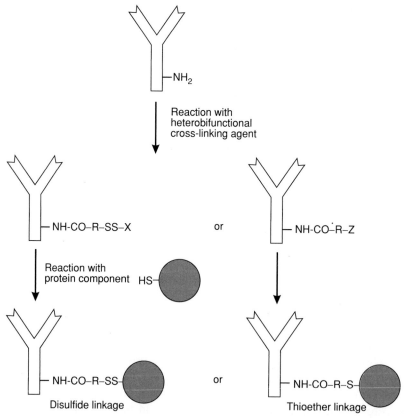

Figure 2.11: Synthesis of antibody–protein conjugates by chemical cross-linking.

–NH–CO–R–SS–*Protein*. Alternatively, the antibody component may be substituted with an alkylating group, *Antibody*–NH–CO–R–Z, and reacted with *Protein*–SH to form a stable thioether-linked conjugate: *Antibody*–NH–CO–R–S–*Protein*.

The covalent modification of Lys residues is heterogeneous with regard to the number of cross-linker molecules introduced per antibody molecule and the locations of the substituted aa residues. Following chemical conjugation of an antibody molecule to another protein, the reaction mixture usually contains conjugate molecules of heterogeneous structure and unconjugated molecules of each component. Purification procedures are necessary to remove unreacted components and to resolve singly or multiply substituted conjugate molecules. Conjugation of a relatively large protein molecule to an antibody can alter the properties of either one or both components unpredictably, depending upon the sites on the molecules at which cross-linking occurs. In some instances, it is possible to use genetically engineered components to create immuno-conjugate molecules of homogeneous structure by site-specific attachment, and so minimize the risk of functional impairment upon conjugation.

2.7 Genetically engineered antibodies

2.7.1 Mutant Mabs

The genetic manipulation of Ig-gene structure by site-directed mutagenesis (sdm), combined with the expression and assembly of recombinant Ig chains in appropriate cell types, allows the production of novel antibody molecules with optimized properties. One application involves the introduction of Cys residues into precisely selected sites in Ig molecules to enable chemical modification and conjugation. The placement of a single additional Cys residue in the C_H3 domain at the C-terminus of a γ chain results in the formation of a novel inter-molecular disulfide bond and converts a monomeric IgG into a tail-to-tail Mab dimer. In another example, the C_H1 domain of an IgG Mab was modified by the introduction of a single Cys residue without adverse effect upon its antigen-binding properties. The thiol group of this Cys residue functioned as the site for the chemical attachment of a ligand. Another application involves the alteration of key aa residues to eliminate antibody effector functions. The replacement of the unique aa residue that is the site of Asn-linked glycosylation in the C_H2 domains of IgG Mabs makes carbohydrate addition during H chain synthesis impossible (Section 1.3.6). Aglycosyl IgGs bind only weakly to Fcγ receptors and cannot effectively activate Fcγ receptor-bearing immune effector cells. Alternatively, the ability to bind to effector cells can be abrogated by introducing aa substitutions that directly incapacitate the Fcγ receptor-binding site of the antibody (Section 1.6.2).

More extensive alteration to antibody structure, such as the deletion or substitution of entire Ig domains, is possible by exploiting the exon structure of Ig genes. Domain deletion can be used to eliminate completely the C_H2 domains of an IgG Mab. One such C_H2 domain-deleted Mab (125 kDa approx.) retained the antigen-binding characteristics of the parent Mab but lacked the capacity to activate immune effectors and exhibited more rapid clearance from the circulation than the parent Mab (Section 1.6.3).

2.7.2 Bivalent antibody fragments

New antibody-like molecules can be constructed by recombination of Ig domains in novel orientations. Recombinant antibody fragments, such as Fab and scFv fragments, are generally expressed by *E. coli* as univalent antigen-binding proteins (Section 2.5.2). Bivalent antibody fragments can be obtained in a number of ways (*Figure 2.12*). F(ab')₂

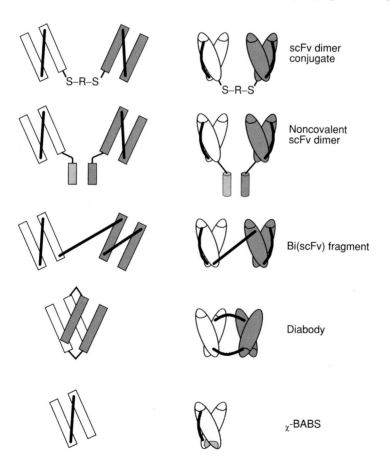

Figure 2.12: Structure of bivalent single-chain Fv antibodies.

fragments can form in *E. coli* by the spontaneous dimerization of recombinant Fab′ fragments via disulfide bond formation. Alternatively, single Cys residues can be introduced at the carboxy-termini of recombinant Fab or Fv proteins to permit dimer formation by means of chemical cross-linking procedures (Section 2.6.2). Bivalent proteins consisting of Fab dimers or scFv dimers, which have been termed mini-antibodies, can be produced directly in *E. coli* by genetically fusing the antibody domains, via a flexible peptide hinge, to several types of polypeptide that form amphipathic helices (Section 2.7.3). Bispecific recombinant Fab dimers can be expressed in *E. coli* by genetically linking two different Fab molecules to discrete leucine zipper structures. The leucine zipper polypeptide domains used are derived from the *fos* and *jun* oncogene products that associate naturally to form noncovalent heterodimers. Furthermore, Cys residues can be incorporated at the carboxy-terminal ends of the dimerizing polypeptides to encourage the formation of a disulfide linkage between the associated Ig chain–leucine zipper fusion proteins.

Bispecific scFv proteins can be produced by one of three approaches (*Figure 2.12*). The first is to genetically link together two scFv fragments into a single-chain recombinant bi(scFv) by means of a long polypeptide linker that spans the distance between the carboxy-terminus of one scFv fragment and the amino-terminus of the other without interfering with the antigen-combining site of either fragment. A second strategy is based on the observation that purified scFv monomers form noncovalent dimers at high concentration by an interaction between the V_H and V_L domains of different monomers. When the V_H and V_L domains from antibodies A and B are fused into $V_HA–V_LB$ and $V_HB–V_LA$ 'cross-over' combinations by a short linker peptide, the pairing of domains present within the same chain is prevented. Upon co-expression, however, the two chains associate noncovalently to form heterodimers instead. The heterodimeric proteins, which have been termed diabodies, contain two functional antigen-combining sites (*Figure 2.12*). Finally, novel antigen-binding properties can be introduced into scFv molecules directly. Chimeric bispecific antibody binding sites (χ-BABS) are formed by the incorporation of CDR loops from a second Mab molecule into the parts of the scFv molecule that normally interact with the C_H1 or C_L domains in the parent Mab and are located at the opposite end of the molecule to the natural antigen-combining site of the scFv.

In the same way that the V_H and V_L domains, which constitute the antigen-combining site of antibody, can be linked genetically to form univalent or bivalent scFv fragments, antigen-binding scFv and bi(scFv) fragments can be linked genetically to human C region domains. Ig-like chains expressed from scFv protein–hinge–C region gene fusions in transfectoma cell lines can assemble into antibody-like dimers that retain the antigen-binding characteristics of the V regions and the effector functions mediated by the C region.

2.7.3 Antibody fusion proteins

Entirely novel functions can be introduced into antibody molecules by fusing gene segments that encode Ig chains with genes that encode non-Ig polypeptides. Antibody–protein fusion at the genetic level is an attractive approach to introducing non-Ig components because a precise site-specific ligation between two components is achieved without the need for the complicated chemical modification and purification procedures employed in the synthesis of antibody–protein conjugates (Section 2.6.3). However, the success of the approach is dependent upon the ability of the individual components of the fusion product to fold independently and to reconstitute functional domains in the appropriate expression system.

Protein fusion partners for Ig chains include enzymes, toxins, growth factors, cytokines and the extracellular domains of membrane surface antigens. Such proteins can be fused genetically to the carboxy-terminal end of the intact H chain or to truncated H chains lacking one or more C domains, so that the resultant antibody molecules retain their natural antigen-combining capacity and are endowed with novel effector functions. Conversely, the V domains can be replaced with non-Ig ligands to create antibody-like molecules that possess novel antigen-binding specificities yet retains the natural antibody effector functions (Section 3.5.3). Finally, it is possible to create functional fusion proteins that comprise three components – a ligand domain, an Ig domain and an effector domain – within a single recombinant polypeptide chain.

2.8 Phage antibodies

Key elements of the natural immune system (Sections 1.4 and 1.5) can be imitated *ex vivo* by using genetic engineering methods to express recombinant Ig molecules in experimental biological systems. Antibody fragments, such as Fab and scFv, may be expressed directly on the surface of eukaryotic cells, bacteria and viruses as genetic fusions with transmembrane anchors, outer membrane proteins or coat proteins, respectively. The most efficient and successful systems to date employ bacteriophages that infect and replicate in *E. coli*, such as λ phage and, especially, nonlytic filamentous phages such as M13 or fd. Antigen-selective phage antibodies can be identified by means of binding, the selected phage amplified and the genes encoding the antigen-specific V domains isolated.

2.8.1 Phage display of antibody fragments

The first objective of an artificial expression system is to provide a means by which the display of antibody with particular antigen-binding specificity is linked to the expression of the genes encoding the antibody, by analogy with the B lymphocyte cell that contains uniquely rearranged Ig genes specifying a single idiotype (Section 1.5).

The filamentous phages consist of long, thin virions in which a single-stranded DNA genome is encapsulated within a protein coat. The major coat protein, pVIII, is present on the surface of wild-type (wt) phage in approximately 2700 copies and forms the body of the virion coat. A minor coat protein, pIII, is present in 3–5 copies located at one tip of the phage particle. Both pIII and pVIII are synthesized with signal sequences that direct their transport to the inner membrane of the bacterium where the signal sequence is proteolytically cleaved to release the mature protein in the periplasmic space ready for virion assembly. Ig molecules that are known to fold correctly in the periplasm, including L and Fd chains and scFv fragments (Section 2.5.2), may be fused genetically to either pIII or pVIII and expressed as functional antigen-binding domains on the surface of the phage (*Figure 2.13*).

The pIII coat protein comprises two domains. The carboxy-terminal domain anchors pIII to the phage coat. The larger amino-terminal domain forms a knob-like structure projecting away from the phage that binds to F pili of *E. coli* in the course of infection (*Figure 2.13*). The intact pIII molecule can tolerate the addition of Ig domains to the amino-terminal domain without loss of infectivity. If the amino-terminal domain is excised and Ig domains are fused to the carboxy-terminal domain instead, the resultant phage is not by itself infective. In this case, infectivity can be restored by binding wt pIII to the surface of the virion via the target antigen (Section 2.8.3). Alternatively *E. coli* can be co-infected with a phagemid, a bacterial plasmid that contains a phage origin of replication, to encode the wt pIII. Competition between wt pIII and pIII–Ig chain fusions for assembly into virions results in populations of phage that predominantly contain a single pIII–Ig chain fusion protein and are therefore mostly univalent. Fusion of Ig domains to the pVIII protein disrupts virion assembly and so wt pVIII must always be supplied via a phagemid. The resultant recombinant phages display multiple copies of the pVIII–Ig chain fusion protein on the particle surface and are therefore multivalent. In each case, the recombinant phage particle contains a copy of the viral genome that encodes the specific coat protein–Ig chain fusion protein expressed on the virion surface.

2.8.2 V domain repertoire cloning

The second requirement of an artificial system that mimics production of antibody by the immune system is a source of V-domain gene diver-

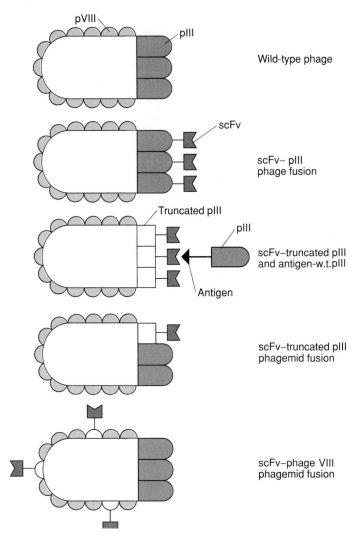

Figure 2.13: Display of antigen-binding antibody fragments on phage.

sity (Section 1.5.4) and cloning procedures that allow the random assortment and combination of V_H- and V_L-domain genes to create a repertoire of antigen-binding fragments (*Figure 2.14*).

Libraries of cloned V-domain gene combinations introduced into the phage expression system have been derived from a number of different sources.

Biased combinatorial libraries. Obtained from animals following immunization, or from humans who have mounted an immune response to infection or vaccination, the V-domain genes in this kind of library

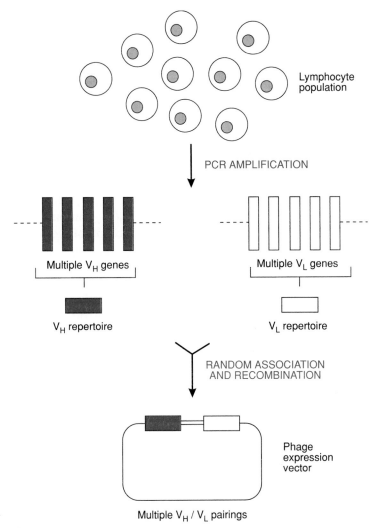

Figure 2.14: Combinatorial linkage of V_H- and V_L-gene libraries.

are derived predominantly from hyperimmune lymphocytes and consequently the library is biased in its usage of V_H- and V_L-domain genes.

Naïve combinatorial libraries. Derived from peripheral blood lymphocytes or bone marrow cells in the absence of specific immunization, the V-domain genes in a naïve library generally reflect the natural repertoire of genes in lymphocytes that have not been subjected to the mechanisms of antigen-driven proliferation and clonal selection that bias gene usage in immunized animals.

Semi-synthetic combinatorial libraries. Created by combining portions of natural V genes that have not undergone rearrangement with randomized synthetic gene sequences encoding the HR3 of the V_H and V_L domains, semi-synthetic gene libraries are designed to include a wider diversity of gene sequences than is present in the native repertoire.

Biased combinatorial libraries are useful for identifying V_H/V_L combinations that specify high-affinity antigen-binding fragments recognizing a particular immunogen. In the case of combinatorial libraries derived from mixed immune lymphocyte populations, the actual pairings of V_H- and V_L-domain genes from hyperimmune cells become scrambled by the cloning procedures and the native V_H/V_L combinations are not necessarily recovered. Non-natural V_H/V_L combinations may none the less generate antibody fragments of acceptable antigen-binding affinity and specificity. The original V_H/V_L pairings can be retained by using PCR methods that amplify and link the V_H and V_L domain genes present within individual cells. The purpose of creating naïve or semi-synthetic libraries is to provide a more extensive source of V-domain gene diversity. Antibody fragments capable of binding to a range of different antigens can be produced by the random combination of V_H- and V_L-domain genes from such libraries. Even high-affinity antibody fragments can, in principle, be identified directly from naïve combinatorial libraries, provided that the repertoire of V_H/V_L combinations is sufficiently large.

2.8.3 Selection of phage antibody

A third essential component of an artificial immune system is a procedure that mimics the natural process by which the binding of antigen drives the clonal expansion of antigen-specific B cells and thereby increases the prevalence of the V-domain genes that encode the antigen-combining site of the surface Ig.

Phage antibodies with affinity for a particular antigen can be identified by *in vitro* screening assays. Target antigen-specific phage present within a library of phage particles that bear different antibody fragments with diverse antigen-binding specificities can be purified rapidly by several cycles of binding to target antigen, elution, infection and replication. Selection by this approach results in the multiplication and enrichment of a unique type of antigen-binding phage (*Figure 2.15*). In an alternative approach to phage selection, the processes of antigen recognition and bacterial infection are linked so that the enrichment of antigen-specific phage from a population of phage with multiple antigen-binding specificities is based upon preferential antigen-selected replication rather than physical separation. Phage that express carboxy-terminal domain pIII–Ig chain fusions, and which therefore lack the

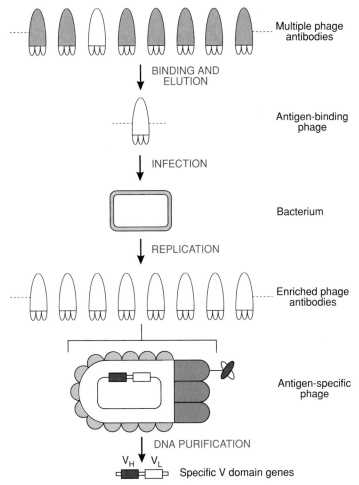

Figure 2.15: Selection of antigen-specific phage antibody.

ability to infect bacteria (Section 2.8.1), can have their infectivity restored if they bind via the displayed antibody fragments to a conjugate or fusion protein comprising the target antigen linked to a wt pIII protein. Attachment of wt pIII to the surface of an antigen-specific phage particle enables it to infect the bacterium and undergo replication.

2.8.4 Affinity maturation of phage antibody

A fourth desirable feature of an artificial immune system is that it should be possible to subject the V_H- and V_L-domain genes identified by phage selection procedures to mutational procedures able to create variant phage antibodies in a process that mimics affinity maturation (Section 1.5.5).

The antibody fragments that are selected by screening naïve or semi-synthetic combinatorial gene libraries using phage expression are most likely to be of low antigen-binding affinity because the V-domain genes in the library have not undergone the process of affinity maturation in the animal. The initial antigen-selected V-domain gene pool can be mutated by a number of different methods.

Random mutagenesis. Random mutations may be induced *in vitro* during PCR amplification by the use of error-prone polymerase, a high number of amplification cycles, biased ratios of nucleotide triphosphates or spiked oligonucleotide primers. Another approach is to use strains of bacteria that introduce mutations into recombinant genes *in vivo*. Several repeated rounds of mutation and selection are generally necessary to generate and propagate phage antibodies with optimized affinity.

Codon-based mutagenesis. The approach selectively targets mutations to the regions of the V-domain genes encoding the HRs which are known to accumulate mutations preferentially during the natural process of affinity maturation. Codon-based mutagenesis replaces entire nucleotide triplets rather than single nucleotides and generates diverse libraries that contain V-domain genes with CDR segments randomized for the 20 possible aa residues at each position.

Chain shuffling. The ability to manipulate V_H- and V_L-domain gene libraries separately allows the diversity of such libraries to be more fully explored once genes encoding a low-affinity antibody fragment have been cloned. The V_H-domain gene isolated from an antigen-selected phage is first paired with all the V_L-domain genes in the repertoire by cloning. Phage antibody with improved affinity for the target antigen is selected and the V_L-domain gene identified. The new V_L-domain gene is then, in turn, combined with the entire V_H-domain gene repertoire and subjected to a second screening cycle to identify phage antibody with even higher affinity.

2.8.5 Human antibodies by repertoire cloning

Human antibody fragments can be derived from phage repertoires by several routes. The first involves the identification of phage antibodies encoded by repertoires of V-domain genes isolated from the B lymphocytes of infected or vaccinated humans. This approach allows the identification of high-affinity antibody fragments recognizing foreign antigens. The second route is to screen phage antibody repertoires encoded by naïve combinatorial libraries derived from unimmunized human cells. The approach has the potential advantage that it can generate human antibody fragments that are capable of recognizing self as well as non-self antigens and that would otherwise be impossible to produce by con-

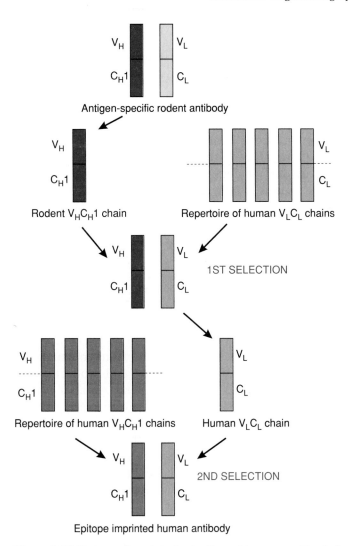

Figure 2.16: Epitope-imprinted selection of human antibody by chain shuffling.

ventional immunization. A third method, called epitope imprinted selection, starts with a rodent antibody of known target antigen specificity and uses chain shuffling (Section 2.8.4) to direct the selection of an equivalent human antibody fragment (*Figure 2.16*). The rodent V_H-domain gene is first combined with a human V_L-domain gene repertoire and phage antibody that is able to bind the target antigen is isolated. The human V_L-domain gene selected is then combined with a human V_H-domain gene repertoire and a second step of selection is used to identify a fully human antibody fragment with the same epitope specificity as the original rodent antibody.

2.9 Catalytic Mabs

Enzymes are able to catalyze chemical transformations by forming a complex with substrate and lowering the activation energy of the reaction. The structure of the enzyme active site is complementary to that of the highly unstable transition state of the reaction. In principle, Mabs should also be capable of catalyzing chemical reactions provided that the structure of the antigen-combining site is complementary to that of the transition state. In practice, Mabs that have been raised against chemically stable structural analogs of reaction transition states do indeed exhibit catalysis and resemble conventional enzymes in terms of features such as substrate specificity and stereoselectivity. Although the catalytic rates of catalytic Mabs, also termed abzymes, can approach those of naturally occurring enzymes, they are generally lower by several orders of magnitude.

Novel catalytic Mabs can be created by using sdm to introduce particular aa residues with side-chains that are involved in catalysis directly into the antigen-combining site. Similar procedures can introduce metal co-ordination sites, useful because metal ions are important co-factors in a large number of enzyme-catalyzed reactions. Alternatively, antibody fragments with catalytic properties can be selected from combinatorial libraries by using screening methods that detect the end-products of the catalyzed reaction on a preselected substrate *in vitro*. Another type of selection assay involves the use of genetic mutants of bacteria or yeast that lack an enzyme activity upon which cell growth or survival depends. Cells expressing intracellular antibody fragments that catalyze a similar reaction to the missing enzyme have a growth advantage on an appropriate selection medium and can therefore be identified. Random mutagenesis combined with rounds of screening and selection may succeed in generating catalytic Mabs with optimized activity.

Chapter 3

Strategies in antibody therapy

3.1 Introduction

Strategies for antibody therapy involve a number of different ways of exploiting the unique molecular properties of Ig molecules. Antibody binding via the Fab arms can block the action of soluble signaling factors, cellular receptors and microbial surface antigens. Intact Ig molecules can stimulate the effector arm of the immune system via the Fc region at target sites selected by the antigen-combining sites of the antibody. Antibodies may also exert immune-regulatory effects either by direct binding to antigens on cells of the immune system or through the anti-idiotypic network. Conventional polyclonal Igs and Mabs are not guaranteed to activate natural immune effector systems efficiently with the potency required to control disease. Antibody can be used instead to target agents that are potent stimulators of different immune mechanisms. Antibodies can also be used to target cytotoxic agents such as radionuclides, chemotherapeutic drugs and naturally occurring protein toxins, or drug delivery vehicles such as liposomes that can be loaded with cytotoxic agents. Immunoconjugates or fusion proteins with toxic entities have highly potent cytotoxic effects but also exert toxic side-effects on normal tissues. The therapeutic efficacy of drug targeting can be improved by separating the processes of antibody localization at the target site and delivery of the cytotoxic agent into separate phases. Finally, antibody technology has potential value in gene therapy, either as a means of targeting viral or nonviral DNA vectors, or as the product of gene expression to interfere with or to redirect cellular function.

3.2 Principles of antibody therapy

Antibodies can interfere with the function of molecules, cells and organisms that are involved with disease in three different ways. First, antibodies can neutralize the action of soluble or cell-associated molecules by simply binding to them directly (Section 3.3). Secondly, antibodies can engage and stimulate natural protective mechanisms, principally elements of the immune system, to induce selective control or destruction of target cells (Sections 3.4 and 3.5). Thirdly, antibodies can be used to target agents that kill cells directly, alter their behavior or serve to enhance the action of other therapeutic protocols (Sections 3.6–3.8).

Four properties of antibody molecules are especially relevant to antibody therapy:

Binding function. The selective binding ability of antibodies, which resides in the structure of the V regions, allows Ig molecules to identify abnormal and disease-related molecules or cells and distinguish them from their normal and healthy counterparts.

Effector function. The ability to interact with other components of the immune system, via molecular interactions mediated by the Fc region, can enhance the potency of action of antibodies that recognize target antigens on cells.

Immune-regulatory capacity. The unique three-dimensional structure of the antigen-combining site, the idiotypic region, is capable of stimulating specific regulatory immune responses by binding directly to antigens on immune cells and stimulating the anti-idiotypic network.

Carrier function. The relatively long half-life of antibody in the circulation, a function both of the molecular size of Ig and the properties of the Fc region, enhances the duration of antibody effects *in vivo*.

Natural antibodies, or recombinant Mabs of conventional Ig structure, may be appropriate and effective agents for therapy of human disease. The molecular engineering of Mabs, by which Ig domains can be modified, eliminated or recombined (Sections 2.4 and 2.5), allows the selection of natural Ig functions to optimize the properties of the therapeutic Mab according to the characteristics of the disease target (Chapter 4). Structural variations are generally introduced either to improve upon the poor efficacy of conventional antibodies or to minimize the side-effects occasioned by unwanted interactions with regions of the antibody that are not essential to their therapeutic action (Sections 2.7.1 and 2.7.2). The conjugation or genetic fusion of antibodies and antibody fragments with other agents that exert biological effects (Sections 2.6 and 2.7.3) can be used either to replace or to augment the natural functions of the Ig molecule.

3.3 Blockade of molecular function

3.3.1 Antibodies

Antibody molecules can bind to foreign substances, such as natural poisons or synthetic drugs, and neutralize their toxic actions within the

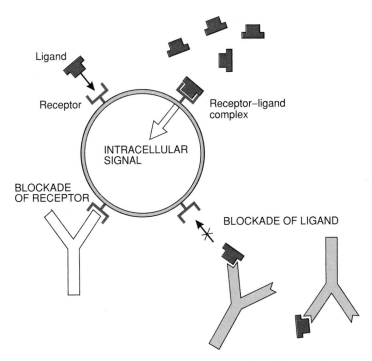

Figure 3.1: Antibody blockade of receptor–ligand interactions.

body. Similarly, antibodies that bind to soluble mediators, growth factors or cytokines can block the ability of these signaling molecules to interact with their cognate cellular receptors and so prevent their biological actions. Alternatively, antibodies that block the ligand binding sites on cellular receptors can prevent the triggering action of soluble ligands (*Figure 3.1*). Antibodies directed against certain epitopes on receptor molecules can desensitize a cell to the presence of the ligand by decreasing the affinity of the receptor for its ligand or by triggering the down-regulation of the receptor by internalization. The function of other types of cell surface antigen, such as enzymes and adhesion molecules, can also be blocked by antibody. Blockade of the surface antigens of viruses and bacteria can interfere with their ability to interact with the receptor molecules by which they adhere to and enter into target cells within the body.

The attraction of antibody blockade as a therapeutic strategy is that simple screening for strong antigen binding selects antibodies with neutralizing properties in the form of either intact Ig or antigen-binding fragments. The success of the approach depends on how effectively the pathogenic action of the target antigen is abrogated. Therapeutic efficacy is a function of the amount of antibody that can be administered, its ability to reach the target site, how strongly the antibody binds the antigen and the capacity of the body to clear the immune complexes formed without side-effect. In acute conditions, where the target antigen is likely to be present only transiently, a short-term treatment with antibody can be highly effective provided that the antigen is largely neutralized. If the target antigen is continuously regenerated in the course of a disease, repeated treatment with antibody may be essential. Thus, in chronic disorders, antibody blockade may ameliorate the effects of the disease without actually addressing its underlying cause, although this approach can achieve significant therapeutic benefit in appropriate clinical circumstances.

3.3.2 Immunoadhesins

An immunoadhesin is a hybrid molecule comprising all or part of a non-Ig adhesive protein molecule genetically linked to antibody C domains (Section 2.7.3). By analogy with antibodies, immunoadhesins are bivalent molecules in which the antigen-binding Fab arms have been replaced with the soluble ligand-binding portion of a cell-surface receptor that is capable of binding a soluble or cell-associated ligand with natural specificity and affinity (*Figure 3.2*). The adhesive portion of such constructs competes directly with endogenous cellular receptors for binding of the ligand. The inclusion of the antibody Fc region endows the fusion protein with a longer circulating half-life (Section 1.6.3) and so a longer duration of action than the soluble receptor itself. The Fc region of the immunoadhesin may additionally mediate the activation of immune effector cells (Sections 1.6.1 and 1.6.2).

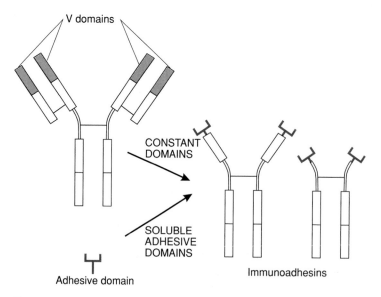

Figure 3.2: Molecular structure of immunoadhesins.

3.4 Immune activation

Antibodies that interfere with the biological function of cells by blocking the action of key cell-surface antigens are generally cytostatic. In
clinical situations where the targeted elimination of invading micro-
organisms or human cells involved in disease is desirable, the ability of
antibodies to harness the powerful cell-killing capacity of the immune
system is advantageous (Section 1.6). The ability of Ig molecules to stimulate immune effector mechanisms resides in the Fc region. One strategy involves the use of natural antibody molecules or antibodies that
have been manipulated to enhance their interaction with human
immune effectors (Section 3.4.1). A second approach, known as effector
cell retargeting, uses antibody derivatives that combine different V
regions recognizing both target and immune effector cells (Section
3.4.2). A third approach seeks to improve upon the natural properties of
the antibody molecule by combining it with agents that are potentially
capable of more potent activation or that can engage the immune
system in a different way (Section 3.4.3).

3.4.1 Antibodies and antibody derivatives

Antibodies can promote complement activation, phagocytosis, or
ADCC (Sections 1.6.1 and 1.6.2). The capacity of an antibody molecule
to stimulate these immune effector mechanisms is a function of both its
structure and the manner of its binding to the target antigen at the
cell surface. Polyclonal Ig contains a mixture of antibody isotypes and
target antigen specificities and so is capable of a spectrum of immune-
activating effects that may adequately mimic natural immunity. On the
other hand, Mabs have a single target specificity and isotype. In practice,
the precise immune-activating effects of individual Mabs may be quite
weak or, conversely, may exceed those that can be achieved with polyclonal antibodies. The relevance of the different immune effector
mechanisms in combating disease is not fully understood and so the production of effective Mabs has often been a matter of trial and error
rather than one of rational design. Nevertheless, it has proven worth-
while to pursue a number of approaches (*Table 3.1*).

Monomeric antibody. Rodent Mabs with appropriate IgG isotypes can
activate human complement and bind with high affinity to Fcγ receptors
on cells of the human immune system (Section 2.3.2). Alternatively,
human Mabs (Sections 2.3.3 and 2.3.4) or recombinant rodent/human
chimeric and humanized Mabs (Section 2.4) can be employed. Further
modifications can be achieved by genetic manipulation to switch,
eliminate or duplicate domains of different isotypes or to introduce
site-specific changes in order to influence the activation of effector
functions (Section 2.7.1).

Table 3.1: Antibodies and derivatives for immune activation

Class	Type	Properties
Monomeric antibody	Polyclonal Monoclonal Chimeric Human(ized)	Bivalent binding Fc-mediated immune activation
Dimeric antibody	Cross-linked Recombinant	Multivalent binding Enhanced immune activation
Engineered derivatives	Bispecific Mab Fab/c fragment Fab′-IgG conjugate Fab′-Fc conjugate	Univalent binding Fc-mediated immune activation
	Fab′-Fc$_2$ bis Fab′-Fc	Univalent/enhanced activation Bivalent/enhanced activation
Hybrid fusion proteins	Ligand–Ig C domains	Bivalent binding Fc-mediated immune activation

Dimeric antibody. The immune-activating effects of antibodies can be substantially enhanced, in some cases, by increasing their binding to the cell surface and their ability to bind complement or Fcγ receptors through multivalent interactions. Dimeric Mabs possess a higher avidity of binding because of the increased number of antigen-combining sites and can be better activators of immune effectors because the two Fc regions are juxtaposed within a single molecule. Antibody dimers can be produced by means of chemical cross-linking procedures (Section 2.6) or by using sdm to introduce a novel inter-molecular disulfide bond between the H chains of two antibody molecules (Section 2.7.1).

Engineered derivatives. Enhanced avidity of binding to target cells is not always an advantage in immune activation. The cross-linking of antigens on the cell surface by bivalent Mabs can induce antigenic modulation and result in the removal of the bound Mab by an internalization process (Section 1.6.1). The simplest strategies to circumvent modulation involve antibody molecules with a single combining site for the target antigen, such as univalent Mabs (Section 2.3.3) or Fab/c fragments (Section 2.5.1). A variety of univalent or bivalent Mab derivatives can be constructed by chemically recombining isolated Fab′ fragments with hinge-containing Fc fragments (Section 2.6.2). Enhanced immune activation can be achieved by creating derivatives that contain two Fc regions within a single molecule, by analogy with dimeric antibodies.

Hybrid fusion proteins. Immunoadhesins or immunoligands, which comprise a non-Ig receptor or ligand respectively in place of the antibody V regions, are capable of selectively recognizing cell surface molecules present on target cells and engaging the immune system via the Fc region of the Ig portion of the fusion protein (Section 3.5.2).

3.4.2 Effector cell retargeting

The cytotoxic action of immune effector cells may be directed against cellular targets selected by means of bispecific antibody derivatives. In a bispecific construct, one arm of the antibody is specific for an antigen on the target cell while the other arm is specific for a cell-surface antigen of the effector cell. The cell retargeting action of bispecific constructs is therefore independent of the sites in the Fc region that trigger natural effector functions (Sections 1.6.1 and 1.6.2). Bispecific antibody molecules form multiple bridges between the target and effector cells and can retarget the action of the effector cells by bringing them into close proximity with the target cell (*Figure 3.3*). A variety of antigens on different cell types within the immune system are useful for effector cell retargeting (*Table 3.2*).

Effector cell retargeting using bispecific antibody molecules can bypass the normal antigen specificity and MHC dependence of cytotoxic T lymphocyte action (Section 1.4.3). However, binding and cross-linking is not sufficient to induce cytotoxicity because only certain surface antigens of T cells, such as CD2 and CD3, appear to trigger activation efficiently. Other antigens, such as CD28, do not mediate redirected lysis but enhance CD3-mediated cytotoxicity. The action of retargeted T cells against target cells is highly localized, similar to that of T cells activated

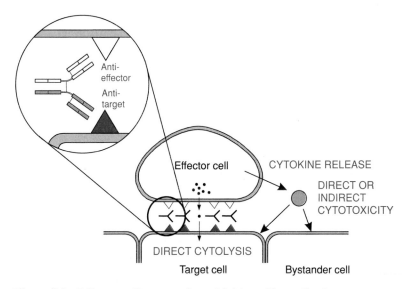

Figure 3.3: Effector cell retargeting with bispecific antibody.

Table 3.2: Target antigens in effector cell retargeting

Antigens	Cell types
T-cell antigens	
TCR/CD3	Cytotoxic T lymphocytes
CD2	Cytotoxic T lymphocytes, NK cells
CD28	Cytotoxic T lymphocytes
Fc receptors	
FcγRI (CD64)	Macrophages
	Monocytes
FcγRIII (CD16)	NK cells
	Macrophages
	Neutrophils

normally through TCR recognition of MHC: peptide complexes. Re-targeted T cells may release inflammatory cytokines, such as TNF-α and IFN-γ, that can exert toxic effects against bystander cells adjacent to, but not in direct contact with, the activated effector cell.

Bispecific antibody molecules can be generated by a number of strategies:

Chemical cross-linking. The simplest approach is to chemically cross-link two Mabs that have the appropriate target and effector cell specificities (Section 2.6.1). However, bispecific Mab heteroconjugates can activate ADCC by means of the Fc regions and thus risk immune destruction of the effector cells themselves.

Bispecific Mabs. Bispecific Mabs derived from quadromas represent a more defined product than Mab heteroconjugates (Section 2.3.3). Moreover, bispecific Mabs can be formed by the combination of parent Mabs with different γ-chain isotypes to generate molecules of mixed isotype that have lost the capacity to bind to Fcγ receptors and to mediate ADCC.

Multimeric Fab′ derivatives. Effector cell retargeting can be achieved with bispecific antibody derivatives consisting of Fab′ fragment dimers that completely lack Fc function (Section 2.6.2). Typically, Fab′ fragments with different antigen specificity are recombined into a bivalent $F(ab')_2$ derivative. Trivalent bispecific $F(ab')_3$ derivatives, in which one Fab′ arm recognizes either the target or effector cell and two Fab′ arms recognize the other cell type, demonstrate improved activity over bivalent derivatives, probably due to the enhanced strength of binding between cells. Trispecific $F(ab')_3$ derivatives that bind to two different surface epitopes or antigens can also activate T cells more effectively than bispecific counterparts that trigger T-cell activation through a single antigen.

Hybrid bispecific derivatives. Effector cell retargeting may be mediated by bispecific constructs in which binding to the target cell occurs by means of a non-Ig ligand connected to the antibody by chemical cross-linking (Section 2.6.3) or genetic fusion (Section 2.7.3).

3.4.3 Antibody conjugates and fusion proteins

The binding selectivity of Mabs or Fab fragments can be used to target agents that activate elements of the immune system by means other than via the interaction with the Fc region of the Ig molecule. A variety of agents has been explored (*Table 3.3*).

Activators of complement. The C3b complement component (Section 1.6.1) can endow Mabs having low or no complement-activating activity with the ability to activate the lytic complement cascade. Cobra venom factor, is a nontoxic glycoprotein that functions similarly to the C3b component during activation of complement can direct complement-mediated killing and stimulate inflammatory reactions at the target site when localized on the surface of a target cell by antibody.

Activators of macrophages. The peptide *N*-formyl-L-methionyl-L-leucyl-L-phenylalanine (fMetLeuPhe) is chemotactic for inflammatory cells such as macrophages and neutrophils. Muramyl dipeptide is a component of the mycobacterial cell wall that stimulates macrophage activity. Antibody delivery of these agents to target cells can, in principle, activate macrophages present at the target site.

Cytokines. Cytokines linked to antibody may have a direct cytotoxic action or can enhance cellular immune effector mechanisms (Section 1.6.2). IFN-α increases the activity of peripheral blood NK cells. TNF-α

Table 3.3: Antibody conjugates and fusion proteins in immune activation

Activating agent	Mechanism of action
C3b complement fragment Cobra venom factor	Activation of complement
fMetLeuPhe Muramyl dipeptide	Attraction or activation of macrophages
IFN-α TNF-α/β IL-2	Stimulation of multiple immune cells
Tuberculin Tetanus toxoid	Activation of antigen-specific inflammatory T cells
Staphylococcal superantigens	Activation of T lymphocyte subfamilies

and TNF-β can induce the expression of MHC antigens and adhesion receptors on target cells, thereby improving immune recognition. IL-2 stimulates T-cell proliferation and T-cell-mediated killing of target cells.

T-cell antigens. The action of inflammatory or cytotoxic T lymphocytes can be directed by the use of Mab to deliver a bacterial protein antigen into target cells. Processing of the antigen and presentation of peptide epitopes in association with MHC molecules at the cell surface can recruit antigen-specific T-cell subsets (Section 1.4.3). T cells recognizing the relevant epitopes are present in the human population that has been immunized with bacillus Calmette–Guerin, or BCG, vaccine or tetanus toxoid.

Bacterial superantigens. T cells can be recruited by antibody targeting of so-called superantigens, such as the exotoxins produced by *Staphylococcus aureus*, that induce immune stimulation by cross-linking MHC class II and TCR molecules (Section 1.4.3). Superantigens bind to MHC molecules at a site lying outside the peptide-binding groove and to the TCR at a site on the Vβ chain outside the antigen-recognition site, thus bypassing the inherent specificity of the system. Antibody–superantigen conjugates therefore stimulate multiple T-cell clones independently of target antigen processing and presentation.

3.4.4 Limitations of immune activation

The therapeutic efficacy of antibody-activated immune mechanisms *in vivo* depends, in part, upon the ability of the antibody, or antibody construct, to localize on the surface of target cells. Premature binding to an excess of effector cells in the circulation may limit the amount of the antibody derivative that reaches target cells unless they are readily accessible. Nonspecific immune activation, leading to complement activation and cytokine release away from the target site, can give rise to side-effects.

A second condition that must be satisfied for the effective action of the immune system is that there must be sufficient numbers of effector cells available for action at the target site. In principle, the numbers of endogenous effector cells in the body can be supplemented by isolating and purifying cells from the blood, activating and expanding them *ex vivo*, and re-infusing them into the patient. The antibody may be administered either concurrently with the infusion of activated effectors or subsequently. Alternatively, effector cells may be recruited and activated *in vivo* by use of relevant cytokines and colony-stimulating factors (Sections 1.4.1 and 1.6.2) before administration of the therapeutic antibody.

Although the immune system can exert highly potent effects against target cells, the system is highly complex and is, of necessity, tightly regulated. In consequence, it may prove difficult to induce selective immune effects of the desired magnitude because the natural response is self-limiting. Indeed, the very existence of some disease states can be taken to reflect an inherent inadequacy of the immune system because a key element in the response has either been rendered ineffective by disease or is lacking altogether.

3.5 Anti-idiotypic vaccination

3.5.1 Anti-idiotypic Mabs

The idiotype of a Mab comprises a cluster of peptide epitopes in, or near to, the antigen-combining site of the molecule (Section 1.3.7). Each Mab has a unique constellation of idiotypic determinants that can provoke an immune response in a recipient. A Mab, typically denoted Ab_1, that is raised against a target antigen can stimulate the production of an anti-idiotypic (anti-id) antibody, or Ab_2, response (*Figure 3.4*). Anti-id antibodies bind with the antigen-combining site of the Ab_1 Mab and a proportion carry a complementary structure, or internal image, that mimics the structure of the target antigen itself. Immunization with an Ab_2 Mab that carries the internal image of the target antigen can, in turn, induce the formation of anti-anti-id, or Ab_3, antibodies that cross-react with the target antigen originally used to raise Ab_1. In other words, a proportion of Ab_3 antibodies will have the same or overlapping antigen specificity as the Ab_1 Mab from which the immunizing anti-id Mab was derived.

Vaccination with anti-id Ab_2 Mab is intended to give rise to an active Ab_3 response that cross-reacts with the target antigen or target cell. This approach has a number of potential advantages. First, anti-id Mabs represent an alternative to vaccination with a natural antigen which may be difficult to prepare safely, reproducibly and in quantity, and which may be poorly immunogenic. Secondly, anti-id Mabs may be able to break immunological tolerance by stimulating silent clones of B cells that are normally suppressed and unresponsive to the natural antigen (Section 1.4.5). Thirdly, anti-id Mabs are capable of stimulating target antigen-specific T-cell responses as well as inducing B-cell production of anti-anti-id Ab_3 antibodies (Section 1.4.6).

3.5.2 Antigenized antibodies

An extension of the anti-idiotypic approach involves molecular engineering of Mabs to replace one or more CDRs of the V domains with peptide epitopes that are based on known antigenic structures

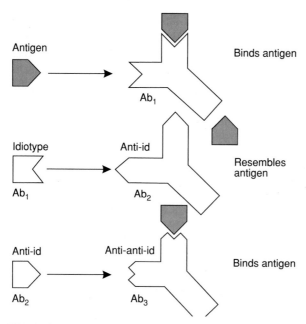

Figure 3.4: Anti-idiotypic antibodies.

derived from target protein antigens. Grafting of the antigenic peptides into the Ig framework imposes conformational restraints that may improve their immunogenicity by comparison with the free unconstrained peptide. 'Antigenized' antibodies have a longer half-life than synthetic peptides and can interact with antigen-presenting cells (APCs), both factors that are likely to enhance humoral and cellular immune responses to the target antigen.

3.5.3 Anti-idiotype fusion proteins

In common with other immunogens, the capacity of the immune system to generate anti-id responses of significant magnitude is enhanced by, if not entirely dependent upon, the use of adjuvants (Section 1.4.4). The reliance upon adjuvants may be circumvented by combining the immunizing Mab with an immune-enhancing cytokine that stimulates antigen presentation and accessory cell functions. A fusion protein comprising Mab and GM-CSF can act as a strong immunogen and produce a good anti-id response without the need for an additional carrier protein or a separate adjuvant.

3.6 Antibody targeting of cytotoxic agents

In circumstances where triggering of the immune system may be insufficient to eliminate disease-causing cells, as in the case of cancer (Section

4.7), antibodies can be employed instead to target the delivery of cyto-toxic agents that act independently of the immune system. Targeted agents are generally either directly toxic to cells or are capable of being converted into toxic entities following successful delivery to the target site. The aim of antibody targeting is to take advantage of the antigen-recognition properties of antibodies to deliver the cytotoxin selectively to target cells and thereby to minimize the degree to which normal cells are exposed to the potentially harmful nonspecific cytotoxic effects of the agent.

3.6.1 Radioimmunoconjugates

Ionizing radiation damages cellular DNA irreparably and kills cells. Radiation therapy can be applied to eliminate disease-related cells either by irradiating the whole body or by more localized treatment. In the case of total body irradiation, normal tissues as well as the target site become irradiated (*Figure 3.5*). Normal dividing cells, such as the stem cells of the bone marrow and the epithelium of the gastrointestinal (GI) tract, are especially sensitive to the cytotoxic effects of radiation. Localized ther-apy can deliver a higher dose of radiation to a disease site and leave sus-ceptible normal tissues undamaged but risks leaving untreated sites of disease that lie outside the irradiated area. In principle, antibody conju-gates made with radiation-emitting nuclides, known as radioimmuno-conjugates, can localize at sites of disease throughout the body when administered systemically, and can irradiate these sites preferentially over time, thus tending to spare sensitive normal tissues (*Figure 3.5*).

The properties of radioimmunoconjugates are determined by the nature of the targeting antibody, the nature of the radionuclide, and the means by which the two are linked. The radionuclides that are most suit-able for radioimmunotherapy (RAIT) deliver a high dose of radiation and have relatively long half-lives of decay to ensure that a sterilizing dose of radiation is delivered in the vicinity of the target (*Table 3.4*). Radioiodine can be attached to antibody by direct chemical reaction (Section 2.6). Metal ion radionuclides are conjugated with antibody via multi-dentate co-ordinating ligands, or chelators, that form tight non-covalent complexes and can be chemically linked to the antibody.

α-Emitters. α-Particles have high energy that is mostly absorbed by tissues within a range of approximately 40–80 μm, or about one cell diameter. Relatively small amounts of α-emitting radionuclides success-fully localized on the surface of a cell can kill it with high efficiency.

β-Emitters. β-Particles are less energetic than α-particles and are mostly absorbed within path lengths of approximately 0.6–6 mm. Con-

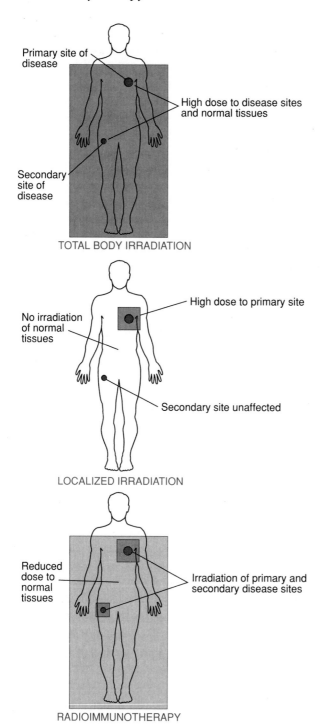

Primary site of
disease

High dose to disease sites
and normal tissues

Secondary
site of
disease

TOTAL BODY IRRADIATION

No irradiation
of normal
tissues

High dose to primary site

Secondary site unaffected

LOCALIZED IRRADIATION

Reduced
dose to
normal
tissues

Irradiation of primary and
secondary disease sites

RADIOIMMUNOTHERAPY

Figure 3.5: Principle of radioimmunotherapy.

Table 3.4: Nuclides for radioimmunotherapy

Radionuclide	Half-life	Energy
α-Particle emitters		
Astatine-211	7.2 hours	5.9 MeV
Bismuth-212 (also β/γ)	1.0 hour	6.1 (8.8) MeV
β-Particle emitters		
Copper-67 (also γ)	2.4 days	0.4, 0.6 MeV
Yttrium-90	2.7 days	2.3 MeV
Iodine-131 (also γ)	8.0 days	0.6, 0.8 MeV
Rhenium-186 (also γ)	3.8 days	1.1 MeV
Auger electron emitters		
Iodine-125 (also γ)	60 days	0.03 MeV

sequently, larger amounts of β-emitting radionuclides must be localized to ensure target cell killing. As β-emitters can exert radiation damage over many cell diameters, they have the potential to sterilize disease cells that are adjacent to the targeted cell but may have failed to bind radioimmunoconjugate either because they lack the target antigen or because of restricted access of the antibody conjugate to the site.

Auger electron-emitters. Nuclides such as Iodine-125 (^{125}I) release low energy Auger electrons that have very short path lengths. To exert cytotoxic effects, these nuclides must be taken up by the cell to ensure close proximity to the nucleus.

The potency of radionuclide targeting is influenced by a number of factors. The dose of radioimmunoconjugate that can localize at target sites is determined, in major part, by the properties of the antibody component of the conjugate. The chemical nature of the radionuclide determines the method by which it is attached to the antibody. Ideally, this linkage should be stable enough to ensure that the maximum dose of active radioimmunoconjugate is delivered to the target. The decay half-life of the radionuclide should be long enough to allow time for the antibody conjugate to localize at the target site and adequately irradiate it. Radiation damage to normal cells occurs from the decay of radioimmunoconjugate that remains in the circulation and perfuses the tissues. The nature of the antibody, radionuclide and linkage influence the metabolism of radioimmunoconjugate, the route of radionuclide excretion and the biodistribution of radionuclide deposition, and so determine the pattern of adverse effects on normal tissues. The side-effects that result from excessive exposure of bone marrow to radiation impose constraints on the amount of radioimmunoconjugate that can be administered systemically (Sections 3.7.1 and 5.5.2).

In another approach, called boron neutron capture therapy, the stable nonradioactive nuclide Boron-10 (^{10}B) is first delivered to the target cell.

Subsequent irradiation with low-energy thermal neutrons, which can penetrate tissue without causing damage, induces conversion of ^{10}B into ^{11}B. The ^{11}B then decays to Lithium-7 (^{7}Li) with the release of an α-particle and γ-radiation. Neutron capture occurs with low efficiency and so relatively large amounts of ^{10}B must be localized for the approach to be effective.

3.6.2 Chemoimmunoconjugates

Chemotherapeutic drugs used in the treatment of cancer act by inhibiting the ability of tumor cells to proliferate (Section 4.7). In consequence, such drugs also affect normal proliferating tissues such as bone marrow and GI epithelium, as well as having the capacity to induce toxic side-effects in other susceptible organs at high doses. A variety of drugs that have different intracellular targets and mechanisms of action have been investigated as candidates for therapeutic immunoconjugates (*Table 3.5*). Many of the common therapeutic agents, or close structural analogs, can be chemically derivatized and reacted with antibody to form covalent linkages (Section 2.6.1). Antibody–drug conjugates, or chemoimmunoconjugates, can exert toxic effects against target antigen-positive cells upon delivering the drug into the cell by means of the antibody component.

In contrast with naked antibody, and antibody conjugates that incorporate either radionuclides or activators of the immune system, which can exert their effects when present at the cell surface, antibody–drug conjugates bound to the surface of a target cell must become internalized to be effective. The drug must become released from the antibody within the cell in a form that retains the capacity to interact with the molecular target (*Figure 3.6*). Internalization of cell-bound chemo-

Table 3.5: Chemotherapeutic drugs for antibody targeting

Class	Drug	Mechanism of action
Alkylating agents	Chlorambucil Melphalan	DNA strand cross-linking
Anti-metabolites	Cytosine arabinoside 5-Fluorodeoxyuridine Methotrexate	Inhibition of DNA or nucleotide precursor synthesis
Plant alkaloids	Vinblastine/vindesine Vincristine	Binding to tubulin and inhibition of mitotic spindle formation
Antibiotics	Doxorubicin/adriamycin Daunorubicin/daunomycin	Intercalation and blockade of DNA synthesis
	Mitomycin C	DNA strand cross-linking
	Bleomycin	DNA cleavage

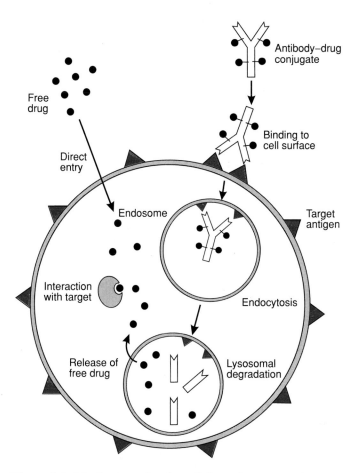

Figure 3.6: Mechanism of action of chemoimmunoconjugates.

immunoconjugate occurs principally by means of endocytosis. Fusion of endocytic vesicles with lysosomes exposes the internalized conjugate to a low pH environment and to a panoply of hydrolytic and proteolytic enzymes. Release of the free drug or active drug derivatives from the antibody component allows penetration to the cytosol. The requirement for antibody-mediated delivery into the cell enhances the selectivity of action of the drug for target cells and can bypass mechanisms of resistance that act by preventing the passage of the drug through the cellular membrane.

The potency of chemoimmunoconjugates depends on a number of factors: the number of conjugate molecules localized at the cell surface, the proportion of antigen–conjugate complexes internalized and the efficiency with which the drug becomes released from the antibody to act on its molecular target. The cytotoxic potency of chemoimmuno-conjugates can be enhanced by a number of maneuvers.

Drug–polymer conjugates. The dose of drug delivered to a target cell can be increased by attaching hundreds of drug molecules to each antibody molecule. Multiple drug molecules are first linked to a bridging molecule that is then chemically attached to an antibody molecule. The bridge may be a protein such as human serum albumin, a carbohydrate such as dextran, or a synthetic peptide polymer such as poly(lysine) or poly(glutamic acid). The approach minimizes the risk of inactivating the antibody by excessive modification (Section 2.6).

Cleavable cross-linkers. The release of drug from internalized conjugate can be enhanced by attaching the drug to the antibody by means of a chemical linkage that is cleaved readily under the conditions found within the lysosome, yet is substantially stable in the extracellular milieu so that drug is not prematurely released from the antibody in the circulation. Chemoimmunoconjugates can be synthesized with acid–labile linkages or with short oligopeptide sequences that are good substrates for lysosomal proteases.

More potent drugs. Antibody–drug conjugates that are effective at lower doses can be made by incorporating analogs of conventional chemotherapeutic drugs with higher potency. Alternatively, highly cytotoxic antibiotics that are obtained from natural sources and have no existing counterparts in the clinic, such as calicheamicin, can be used to create more potent antibody conjugates.

In a different approach, called antibody-directed photolysis, photoimmunotherapy or targeted photodynamic therapy, a nontoxic photosensitizing agent is first targeted to the appropriate site and then irradiated with light of a suitable wavelength. The photosensitizers hematoporphyrin, benzoporphyrin and chlorin e6 release toxic entities such as singlet oxygen ($^1O_2$) that can act both at the cell membrane and within the cell. Relatively large amounts of photosensitizer need to be localized and the target site must be accessible to light either by external irradiation or by use of fiber-optic devices.

3.6.3 Immunotoxins

Immunotoxins are antibody conjugates made with naturally occurring protein toxins or their engineered analogs. Protein toxins of bacterial and plant origin number amongst the most powerful cytotoxic agents known to man. Although the principal toxins – diphtheria toxin, *Pseudomonas* exotoxin and ricin – differ in origin, structure and action, they intoxicate cells by a broadly similar mechanism, dependent upon the co-ordinated action of several portions of the toxin molecule with distinct functions (*Figure 3.7*). Protein toxins contain a discrete polypeptide

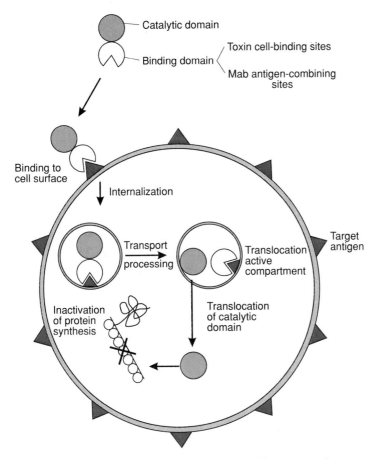

Figure 3.7: Mechanism of action of toxins and immunotoxins.

domain or chain by which they attach to specific cell-surface receptors expressed by the majority of human cell types. The cell-bound toxin becomes internalized via endocytosis or by other routes of uptake determined by the nature of the receptor. A specific catalytic portion of the toxin becomes separated from the binding portion and is then translocated to the cytosol. Finally, the enzyme inactivates the protein synthetic machinery of the cell irreversibly and kills it.

Immunotoxins have a number of potential advantages over antibody conjugates made with chemotherapeutic drugs. Protein toxins have high potency because as few as tens or hundreds of molecules of toxin bound to a cell surface can ensure entry of the single molecule of the enzyme needed to shut down protein synthesis. Consequently, relatively fewer immunotoxin molecules need to localize at the target cell to exert a similar toxic effect to chemoimmunoconjugate. Whereas many chemotherapeutic drugs act against cycling cells, immunotoxins are capable of inactivating resting as well as dividing cells. Moreover, immunotoxins are active against cells that are resistant to the action of conventional drugs because the mechanism of toxin action is quite different. The properties of immunotoxins are determined by the nature of the toxin component.

Toxins and toxin analogs. Antibody–toxin conjugates exert highly potent effects on target cells bearing the antigen recognized by the antibody component but also exhibit nonspecific activity against antigen-negative cells that is mediated by the cell-binding sites of the toxin component. The natural cell-binding sites must be blocked or eliminated to avoid untoward side-effects upon normal tissues. A number of toxin analogs have been developed that have diminished cell-binding capacity yet retain the translocation and catalytic activities of the native toxin (*Table 3.6*). Immunotoxins made either by the stable chemical linkage of toxin analogs to antibody or by genetic fusion of the Ig and toxin components can demonstrate cytotoxic potencies matching the native toxins.

Ricin A chain. An alternative strategy has been applied in the case of ricin, which consists of an active A chain and a binding B chain linked by a single disulfide bond. Ricin A chain can be chemically linked to

Table 3.6: Toxins and toxin analogs for antibody targeting

Toxin	Molecular mass (kDa)	Properties
Diphtheria toxin (DT)	58	Binds to EGF-like receptor ADP-ribosylates elongation factor-2 (EF-2)
DAB 486 (truncated DT)	50	Lack cell binding sites Retain translocation/catalytic function
DAB 389 (truncated DT)	40	
Pseudomonas exotoxin (PE)	66	Binds to α2-macroglobulin receptor ADP-ribosylates EF-2
PE-40 (truncated PE)	40	Lacks cell binding sites Retains translocation/catalytic function
Ricin toxin	64	Binds to galactose-containing cell-surface molecules Specific *N*-glycosidic cleavage of 28S rRNA
Blocked ricin	>64	Cell binding reduced 1000-fold Retains catalytic activity
Ricin A chain	32	Completely lacks cell binding Catalytic chain only
Deglycosylated ricin A chain	32	Chemically modified to destroy mannose/fucose residues
Recombinant ricin A chain	30	Naturally aglycosyl protein

antibody by means of a disulfide bond that mimics the linkage to the B chain in the native toxin. A-chain immunotoxins have high selectivity for target cells because they completely lack the toxin-binding chain. However, in contrast to immunotoxins made with intact ricin, the potency of A-chain immunotoxins varies according to the target antigen. The nature of the antigen determines the route of internalization of the antibody–A chain conjugate and hence its ability to reach the compartments of the cell within which the enzymatically active A chain is released from the antibody and becomes translocated to the cytosol.

A chain analogs. Ricin A chain from native toxin bears oligosaccharide side-chains that divert ricin A-chain immunotoxins to the reticuloendothelial system (RES), and especially the liver. Deglycosylated ricin A chain, prepared by chemical treatment of native A chain, or aglycosyl recombinant ricin A chain made in *E. coli*, are analogs that avoid the carbohydrate-directed cross-reactivity with nontarget tissues. Ribosome-inactivating proteins that resemble ricin A chain, such as saporin or gelonin, can form active immunotoxins when attached to antibody by a disulfide linkage. Human ribonucleases with less specific catalytic action can also be targeted to cells.

A variety of clostridial, staphylococcal and streptococcal bacteria produce cytolytic exotoxins, or cytolysins, that act by mechanisms involving disruption of the cellular membrane rather than interference with some key intracellular function. Cytolysins fall into two general classes: enzymes that hydrolyze membrane phospholipids and proteins that insert into the membrane bilayer, associate together and form pores that disrupt the osmotic stability of the cell. Antibody–cytolysin conjugates, or immunolysins, can mediate antibody-dependent selective cytotoxic effects. The potential advantage of immunolysins, that they can be potently toxic without the need for internalization, is balanced by their capacity to interact with the surface of nontarget cells.

3.6.4 Immunoliposomes

Liposomes are synthetic microscopic vesicles consisting of phospholipid molecules. The phospholipid forms bilayers that mimic cellular membranes in separating an aqueous interior from the external medium. Liposomes can therefore be used to entrap water-soluble agents, such as chemotherapeutic drugs, protein toxins and antisense oligonucleotides, and deliver them to target cells. Interaction of the liposome with the target cell, either by direct fusion with the cellular membrane or by endocytic uptake, delivers the therapeutic agent into the cell (*Figure 3.8*).

The targeting properties of liposomes are influenced by their size and

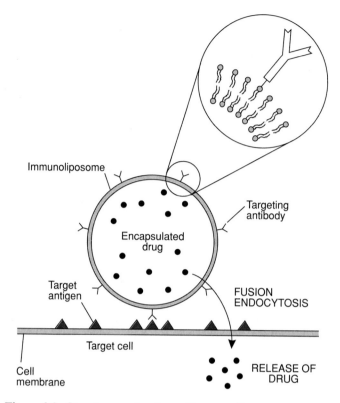

Figure 3.8: Structure and action of immunoliposomes.

lipid composition. Conventional liposomes have the limitations that they are unstable, extravasate only poorly and are subject to rapid clearance by the scavenger cells of the RES. Novel formulations of sterically stabilized, or 'stealth' liposomes, that are less susceptible to RES uptake have prolonged circulation times and enhanced extravasation properties. However, liposomes have no intrinsic selectivity for any particular tissue. The attachment of antibody to the surface of a liposome can direct it to target cells and promote membrane fusion or endocytic uptake. The potential advantage of antibody-targeted liposomes, or immunoliposomes, is the capacity to deliver a higher amount of drug than is possible with conventional antibody conjugates.

3.6.5 Limitations of antibody targeting

Antibody conjugates made by chemical modification procedures are complex to synthesize, purify and characterize (Section 2.6). The carrier function of the antibody molecule can be adversely affected by chemical modification and the attachment of other entities can lead to more rapid clearance from the circulation. In addition, antibody conjugates can be unstable *in vivo*. Radioimmunoconjugates suffer the loss of radionuclide from antibody because of enzymatic deiodination or dissociation of metal ion:chelate complexes. Chemoimmunoconjugates and immunotoxins can break down in the bloodstream if made using the unstable linkages that are incorporated to allow release of the active entity within the target cell (Sections 3.6.2 and 3.6.3). The premature breakdown of active immunoconjugate reduces the dose that can reach the target site and can lead to unwanted and potentially harmful accumulation of the active agent in normal tissues.

The therapeutic efficacy of cytotoxic immunoconjugates and fusion proteins can be limited by the severity of side-effects on nontarget tissues. Radioimmunoconjugates can damage nontarget cells as they circulate throughout the body (Section 3.6.1). In contrast, the internalization of the immunoconjugate molecule is a prerequisite for the cytotoxic action of antibody conjugates incorporating drugs and toxins. However, cells in the vasculature, and in tissues that are readily accessed from the circulation, are continuously exposed to antibody conjugate. Nontarget cells may be sensitive to the potent action of the active agent if the immunoconjugate becomes internalized either by binding to cross-reactive antigen or via nonspecific uptake mechanisms.

3.7 Two-stage targeting approaches

The efficacy of antibody conjugates formed with cytotoxic agents is restricted by toxicity to normal tissues because target and nontarget tissues are simultaneously exposed to the active immunoconjugate (Section 3.6.5). Two-stage approaches to targeting attempt to redress this deficiency by separating the processes of antibody-mediated localization and delivery of the active agent into two phases. The first phase allows time for a nontoxic Mab or immunoconjugate to penetrate tissues and associate with target cells. Following successful localization, the excess unbound antibody may be allowed to clear naturally from the circulation. Alternatively, clearance of the targeting antibody may be intentionally accelerated by the administration of a second agent that binds to it and directs its removal from the bloodstream. In the second phase, the active agent is administered in a form that permits it to interact with the pretargeted Mab or immunoconjugate.

3.7.1 Two-stage radioimmunotherapy

The long circulating half-life of Mabs means that the body is continuously exposed to a background of radiation during the time that a radioimmunoconjugate takes to localize at the target site (Section 3.6.1). The use of antibody fragments with faster rates of clearance from the bloodstream (Sections 2.5.1 and 2.5.2) can reduce the level of background irradiation, but only at the cost of also diminishing the amount of conjugate that accumulates at the target site and hence the radiation dose that is delivered. Higher doses of radiation to the target can be achieved by first localizing the Mab component and then using it to capture a subsequently administered radionuclide conjugate that clears more rapidly from the circulation.

Approaches to two-stage radioimmunotherapy require a capture mechanism such as the interaction between a receptor and its ligand, an enzyme and its active-site inhibitor, or between oligonucleotides of complementary sequence. The best-developed methods have taken advantage of the high-affinity binding interaction between biotin and avidin or streptavidin (*Figure 3.9*). If a Mab–biotin conjugate is first localized at the target site, avidin is used to attach the radionuclide to the immunoconjugate in the second step. In one version, a hapten–radionuclide conjugate chemically linked directly to avidin is administered. In a second

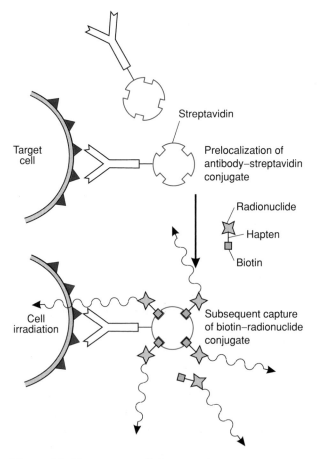

Figure 3.9: Two-stage radioimmunotherapy.

version, unconjugated avidin is first allowed to bind to the localized biotin-immunoconjugate and a hapten derivatized with biotin then carries the radionuclide to the Mab–biotin:avidin complex at the target cell surface. Alternatively, a Mab–streptavidin conjugate can first be localized at the target site and a biotinylated hapten–radionuclide conjugate used in the second step. Biotinylated hapten conjugates have potential advantages for radionuclide delivery because of their small molecular size: they diffuse rapidly into tissues to reach antibody-tagged cells and are rapidly eliminated from the body by excretion through the kidneys, which are relatively radioresistant organs compared with bone marrow. In contrast, avidin is a large protein molecule that penetrates tissues less well and has a significantly longer half-life.

3.7.2 Antibody–enzyme conjugates and fusion proteins

The efficacy of antibody–drug conjugates is limited by the need for a relatively large amount of chemoimmunoconjugate to deliver a cyto-toxic dose to the target cell and efficient internalization of the conjugate (Section 3.6.2). A strategy that circumvents these limitations uses antibody to attach to the surface of the target cell an enzyme that is capable of converting an innocuous substrate, or prodrug, into a toxic agent. This two-step approach, which has been dubbed antibody-directed catalysis or antibody-directed enzyme prodrug therapy (ADEPT), has several potential advantages. First, it allows the pretargeting of the enzyme immunoconjugate or fusion protein to target antigen-bearing cells before the prodrug is administered. Conversion of the prodrug to the active drug then occurs at the sites where immunoconjugate has localized. Secondly, the catalytic activity of the enzyme provides an amplification system able to generate many more molecules of active drug at the target site than could otherwise be delivered by direct chemical attachment of drug to antibody. Thirdly, small active drugs can diffuse rapidly into tissues and exert effects on disease cells that happen to lack the target antigen or are not readily accessible to relatively large molecules of immunoconjugate (*Figure 3.10*).

Chemotherapeutic drugs approved for clinical use, as well as other potent agents, are amenable to chemical conversion into prodrugs that are substrates for a number of well-characterized enzymes (*Table 3.7*). The prodrug should ideally be considerably less toxic than the active drug, and will preferably have a relatively long half-life to ensure that a sufficient dose can reach the target site. The active drug should readily permeate cell membranes and its half-life should be relatively short to minimize the opportunity for it to diffuse away from the target site and affect normal tissues. The prodrug-converting enzyme will ideally be stable *in vivo*, have a high turnover of substrate under physiological conditions, cleave the prodrug hydrolytically to avoid the need for any addi-

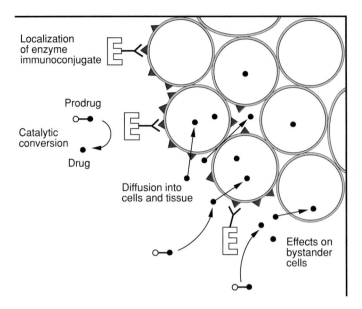

Figure 3.10: Antibody-directed enzyme prodrug therapy.

tional co-factor, and lack any counterpart able to convert the prodrug in normal tissues.

The specificity of targeting using ADEPT is highest when the administration of prodrug is timed to coincide with the maximal accumulation of the antibody–enzyme conjugate at the target site and when the level of conjugate remaining in nontarget tissues or in the circulation is low. Specificity can be further enhanced by inducing the clearance of circulating immunoconjugate once the required amount of enzyme has localized at the target site. One approach is to administer a second Mab that is directed against the enzyme and to which galactosyl residues have been chemically attached. The galactosylated Mab binds to the enzyme immunoconjugate and forms complexes in the circulation that are cleared rapidly via galactose-specific receptors present on parenchymal cells of the liver.

3.7.3 Agent capture with bispecific antibody constructs

Bispecific Mabs or $F(ab')_2$ fragments with dual specificity for the target cell and for an active agent may be used for the first step of targeting, with subsequent administration of the agent and its capture at the target site. Agent capture has been explored with the range of agents that have conventionally been targeted by direct conjugation to antibody, including hapten–radionuclide conjugates, chemotherapeutic drugs, protein toxins, enzymes and cytokines. The approach has the advantage that it

Table 3.7: Systems in antibody-directed enzyme prodrug therapy

Enzyme	Active agent	Substrate
Alkaline phosphatase (calf intestine)	Doxorubicin Etoposide Mitomycin alcohol Phenol mustard	Phosphate derivatives
Carboxypeptidase G2 (*Pseudomonas*)	Benzoic acid mustards	L-Glutamate derivatives
β-Lactamase (bacterial)	Nitrogen mustards Vinblastine analogs	Cephalosporin derivatives
β-Glucuronidase (*E. coli*/human placenta)	Daunorubicin Epirubicin *p*-Hydroxyaniline mustard	Glucuronide derivatives
Penicillin V amidase (*Fusarium*)	Doxorubicin Melphalan	N-(4'-hydroxyphenylacetyl) derivatives
Penicillin G amidase (*E. coli*)	Palytoxin	N-(4'-hydroxyphenylacetyl) derivatives
Cytosine deaminase (yeast)	5-Fluorouracil	5-Fluorocytosine
β-Glucosidase (sweet almond)	Cyanide	Amygdalin

does not require the use of chemical conjugation procedures that can adversely affect the properties of the constituent components of the immunoconjugate (Section 2.6). However, the efficiency with which the active agent localizes depends upon the affinity of its binding to the pretargeted bispecific antibody and its pharmacokinetic properties. In practice, the premixing of the antibody and the agent, rather than a two-phase strategy, may be necessary to ensure the delivery of a satisfactory dose of the agent to the target site.

3.8 Antibody applications in gene therapy

The genetic manipulation of human cells can accomplish the replacement of missing functions in congenital disorders, the introduction of new disease-resistance functions or the induction of cell death. The ability to introduce DNA vectors into target cells by procedures that retain both the function of the therapeutic construct and the viability of the cell is an essential requirement of successful gene therapy. Antibodies have a role to play in determining the selectivity of gene delivery (Sections 3.8.1 and 3.8.2). In addition, cells may be engineered to express antibody domains either intracellularly or on the cell surface (Sections 3.8.3 and 3.8.4).

3.8.1 Immunoviruses

The high efficiency of cellular infection by viruses provides an important means of introducing therapeutic DNA into cells. Viruses combine the ability to package DNA, to bind to the cell surface through viral coat proteins and to release the DNA into the cell by penetration of the endosomal membrane. Recombinant viral vectors have been constructed with retroviruses, adenovirus, adeno-associated virus, vaccinia virus and herpes virus. The value of these vectors for targeting DNA is limited either by restricted cell tropism or by a complete lack of target selectivity. Specific cell transfection can be accomplished with viral vectors *ex vivo*, using target cells that have been isolated and purified, or by delivering the vector directly to the target site *in vivo*. An alternative strategy is to engineer antibody V domains directly on to the surface of viral coat proteins to redirect the target specificity of the vector at the level of cell attachment. 'Immunoviruses' would be expected to retain the ability of the natural virus to package DNA and to deliver it efficiently into the target cell provided that the internalization of the antibody-targeted recombinant virus occurs by a pathway similar to the natural route of viral penetration.

3.8.2 Antifection

'Antifection' is a strategy that uses antibody to target nonviral DNA vectors. In one version, naked DNA is chemically linked directly to the targeting antibody. In another approach, antibody–poly(lysine) conjugates associate noncovalently with DNA. Polycations such as poly(lysine) can complex with the negatively charged DNA molecule and condense it into a compact structure that is more resistant to degradation and better able to enter cells than naked DNA. Antibody–poly(lysine):DNA complexes demonstrate target cell-selectivity dictated by the antigen-binding specificity of the Mab and so antifection may, in principle, be employed for gene therapy. However, synthetic antibody:DNA complexes lack a mechanism of endosomal escape compared with viruses that have become adapted to infect cells efficiently. The inclusion of synthetic peptides to mimic the action of the viral fusogenic proteins that mediate endosomal penetration may enhance the efficiency of antibody-targeted DNA delivery.

3.8.3 Intracellular immunization

Human cells that do not normally express antibodies can be induced to do so by transfection of recombinant Ig gene expression vectors. Ig chains synthesized in the cytosol become translocated normally into the secretory pathway of the cell and assemble into antibody molecules.

Alternatively, antigen-binding fragments of antibody can be retained in the cytosol or directed to intracellular compartments where they are not usually found, such as the nucleus, by appropriate genetic manipulation of signal sequences. The approach has been likened to intracellular immunization because the antibody molecule can bind to and interfere with the action of specific molecular targets within the cell. Potentially, the strategy can inhibit the replication machinery of intracellular parasites or block the function of abnormal cellular products such as mutant oncogene proteins.

3.8.4 Targeting of cytotoxic T lymphocytes

In T-cell immunotherapy, a patient's T lymphocytes are removed, expanded in number and then returned to the patient. T cells can be manipulated further *ex vivo* to enhance their potency and selectivity. One strategy to combine the potent cell-killing activity of cytotoxic T cells with target specificity is to modify T cells genetically so that they express antigen-binding Ig domains on their surface. The resultant 'T-bodies' express hybrid receptors comprising antibody V domains linked to the C domains of the TCR (Section 1.4.3) or TCR-associated subunits involved in signal transduction, and become activated upon binding the target antigen. The approach could, in principle, be extended to different cell-signaling membrane proteins present on other effector cells of the immune system.

3.9 Strategies to improve antibody therapy

3.9.1 Enhancement of antibody localization

Systemic administration by the intravenous (iv) route is the most commonly used means of delivering antibody to the patient. The distribution of antibody between target and nontarget tissues is determined by whether it is given as a short infusion, or bolus, or as a continuous infusion over a longer time period because the pharmacokinetics, or dynamics of distribution, of the administered antibody are influenced by preferential binding to target antigen. Association with the target antigen occurs at a rate that depends upon the concentration of the antibody, its avidity of binding and its ease of access to the target from the bloodstream.

The localization of antibody at less accessible target sites can be enhanced by pre-dosing the patient with a blocking antibody to bind antigen present on molecules or cells in the bloodstream before administering a therapeutic antibody. Alternatively, antibody can be administered by routes other than the iv route to increase the amount that reaches the target site and reduce access to other normal tissues and organs. Antibodies have been successfully administered directly into the pleural, pericardial and peritoneal body cavities, to the liver and brain by intra-arterial routes, to the cerebrospinal space by the intrathecal route and by direct intralesional injection.

The amount of antibody which localizes at a target site that is not readily accessible from the bloodstream is generally only a small fraction of the administered dose because entry into tissues involves distribution through the vascular network, transport across the vascular wall and movement through the interstitium (Section 1.6.3). Physical treatments such as irradiation and hyperthermia applied locally can induce increases in blood flow and vascular permeability at target sites. Alternatively, Mabs can be used as carriers for the delivery of vasoactive cytokines, such as IL-2 and TNF-α, or other substances, such as physaelamin, leukotriene B4, histamine and bradykinin.

3.9.2 Suppression of immune responses

Antibody molecules that are relatively nonimmunogenic in humans can be rendered more immunogenic as a result of chemical modification and the attachment of additional biologically active effectors. Synthetic molecules such as chemical cross-linking agents, metal ion chelators and chemotherapeutic drugs, which do not normally induce immune responses, become the target of an antibody response when conjugated to an antibody carrier. The human immune response is prominent to the non-Ig portion of antibody conjugates or fusion proteins made with non-mammalian proteins and enzymes and, in addition, responses to the Ig component itself may be magnified.

The humoral immune response to antibody or immunoconjugate can be inhibited by co-administering agents, such as cyclosporin A or cyclophosphamide, that broadly suppress the function of T cells and block the ability of the immune system to respond to antigenic stimulation. More selective control of the immune response to soluble antibody may be achieved by using Mabs that interfere with the mechanism of antigen presentation (Sections 1.4.3 and 4.8.4) and thereby induce peripheral tolerance to co-administered antigen. The covalent modification of proteins with the polymer poly(ethyleneglycol), or PEG, has been shown to reduce or abrogate immunogenicity, and PEG conjugates are also capable of inducing tolerance to protein antigens. An antibody–PEG conjugate could, in principle, be used to induce unresponsiveness to an antibody prior to its administration in therapeutic form. Drug immunoconjugates may also selectively suppress the immune response to an administered antibody. If the antibody is conjugated to a cytotoxic drug, B lymphocytes that recognize the antibody and take up the antibody–drug conjugate can be eliminated selectively, while other B cells are left unaffected.

Chapter 4

Target diseases and antigens

4.1 Introduction

Antibodies have found wide application in the detection and diagnosis of disease because of their ability to bind selectively to relevant target antigens. The binding property of antibodies permits the identification of molecules and cells and enables their removal or purification from the blood and other tissues. Antibody therapy began with the exploitation of the discovery that passive administration of serum could transfer immunity to diseases such as diphtheria and tetanus. Antitoxin in the serum was able to neutralize the protein toxins released by the disease-causing bacteria. The neutralizing capacity of antibodies, whether of animal or human origin, makes them useful agents in the treatment of emergency poisoning or infection. The natural protective role of human polyclonal Ig in suppressing viral and bacterial disease is valuable in cases of immune deficiency that arise congenitally or as the result of disease or therapeutic intervention. Antibodies can block the action of the growth factors, cytokines and cellular receptors that are implicated in key pathogenic steps of a broad range of diseases, including bacterial sepsis, cancer, inflammation, autoimmune disease, allergy and wound healing. Antibodies that recognize target antigens on cells involved in disease mechanisms and can block or abolish their function are being explored in the treatment of cancer, inflammatory disease, autoimmune disease, medical complications of organ and tissue transplantation and prevention of ischemia. A number of strategies in antibody therapy, in particular, immune activation and the targeting of cytotoxic agents, are being applied to the treatment of cancer, where the aim is to stop the growth of tumors and eliminate clonogenic tumor cells as completely as possible.

4.2 Diagnostic applications of antibodies

Polyclonal antibodies and Mabs can distinguish between different types of microbe, cell and tissue according to characteristic patterns of antigen expression. Antigen-specific antibodies are used to detect the presence

Table 4.1: Diagnostic applications of antibodies

Method	Purpose	Examples
Ex vivo		
Immunoassay	Identification and quantification of disease markers	Antibodies Cytokines Hormones Liver enzymes Microbial and viral antigens Tumor-associated antigens
Immunocytology	Typing and measuring blood and other cells	Histocompatibility typing CD4/CD8 T-cell ratios
Immunohistology	Identification of cell abnormalities in tissue sections	Pre-cancerous lesions Tumor identification
In vivo		
Immunolocalization	Detection of occult sites of disease in patients	Sites of inflammation Thrombus imaging Tumor metastases

of, and to identify the nature of, microbial infections or the physiological abnormalities that are associated with human disease states. Antibodies recognizing disease-associated antigens are also useful to define the extent of disease, to monitor disease progression and to measure the effectiveness of therapy (*Table 4.1*).

4.2.1 Ex vivo *diagnosis*

In diagnosis, body fluids, cell samples or tissue biopsies are typically removed from patients and reacted with specific antibodies that are linked directly or indirectly to detection systems. Diagnostic systems can be configured in a large variety of ways, depending upon the application and the desired simplicity, speed, sensitivity and accuracy of the assay. Common detection methods involve the use of radiolabels, fluorescent, chemiluminescent or photoluminescent labels, or enzyme-linked chromogenic substrates.

4.2.2 In vivo *diagnosis*

Antibodies may be administered directly to patients to confirm the presence of disease, to identify its location within the body, to gauge its extent and to determine the intensity of therapy. The antibody is generally tagged with an agent that can be detected outside the body. In radioimmunoscintigraphy, a form of radioimmunodiagnosis (RAID), isotopes that emit γ-radiation can be tracked externally using suitable radiation-detecting equipment and imaging procedures. Radionuclides suitable for imaging, commonly Technetium-99m, Indium-111 and Iodine-123, release only γ-radiation and have relatively short half-lives to limit the radiation dose, in contrast with therapeutic radionuclides (Section 3.6.1). Antibodies may also be tagged with nuclides that enable external detection by positron emission tomography scanning. In radioimmunoguided surgery (RIGS), labeled antibodies are administered *in vivo* to localize at disease sites which can then be detected and resected during surgery.

4.3 Therapeutic uses of antibodies *ex vivo*

The ability of antibodies, and especially Mabs, to distinguish between blood cells of different lineage and function by virtue of their characteristic patterns of surface-antigen expression (Section 1.4.1) can be exploited for a number of purposes *ex vivo*. Antibodies may be used either to eliminate specific cell populations involved in disease processes or to purify selected subpopulations of cells intended for therapeutic application (*Table 4.2*).

4.3.1 Cell elimination

In certain clinical situations, notably advanced cancer (Section 4.7), therapeutic protocols are employed that can result in the ablation of the patient's hematopoietic system and so necessitate bone marrow transplantation (bmt) to rescue the patient. In autologous bmt, a portion of the patient's bone marrow is removed before therapy and re-infused after it has been treated *ex vivo* with a tumor-specific Mab in an attempt to eliminate any residual malignant cells. In allogeneic bmt, bone

Table 4.2: Therapeutic uses of antibodies *ex vivo*

Procedure	Target cells	Purpose
Cell elimination		
Transplantation	Tumor cells	Autologous bone marrow purging
	T lymphocytes	Allogeneic bone marrow purging
Cell purification		
Cellular therapy	Stem cells	Blood cell reconstitution
	Cytotoxic T cells	Therapy of viral diseases
	Tumor-infiltrating lymphocytes	Cancer therapy
Gene therapy	T cells/stem cells	Engineered cellular therapy
Diagnosis	Fetal blood cells	Prenatal diagnosis of genetic disease
	Tumor cells	Cancer detection

marrow from a normal donor is infused into the patient after it has been treated *ex vivo* with Mabs specific for T cells to eliminate donor cells that contribute to graft-versus-host disease (GVHD) in the recipient (Section 4.8.6). Generally, Mabs alone are ineffective at cell elimination and are used either in conjunction with complement (Section 1.6.1) or to target cytotoxic agents (Section 3.6). An alternative approach to bone marrow purging is to remove target cells physically, using methods that have been developed for the isolation of specific cell populations (Section 4.3.2).

4.3.2 Cell purification

Antibodies can be used to purify antigenically distinct cells from a mixed population of cell types. Mabs may be used to purify the hematopoietic stem cell fraction, either from the bone marrow or from peripheral blood. Mabs can also positively select T-lymphocyte populations that can be expanded in culture and then returned to the patient for the cellular immunotherapy of cancer and viral infection. In both cases, the purified cell populations may also serve as the target of *ex vivo* gene therapy protocols designed to augment their therapeutic properties (Section 3.8.4). The isolation and purification of antibody-selected cells has been achieved by three different approaches.

Cell panning. Mabs recognizing an antigen on target cells are permanently affixed to the polystyrene surface of disposable culture flasks by covalent attachment. Target cells bind to the immobilized Mab whereas nontarget cells fail to bind, remain in suspension, and are washed out. The captured cells are then dislodged free of the selecting Mab, which remains attached to the flask.

Continuous-flow column. Antigen-specific Mab linked to biotin is added to a mixture of cells in suspension and allowed to bind to the target cells. The suspension is poured rapidly through a column formed of avidin-coated beads. Cells coated with the biotinylated Mab bind tightly whereas uncoated cells pass through the column unretarded. The captured cells are then dislodged from the column and collected.

Magnetic microspheres. The target-specific Mab is attached to microspheres that contain magnetite. The antibody-coated beads and target cells are allowed to associate in suspension. The cellular mixture is then passed through a magnetic field. The beads and bound target cells are retained in the magnet whereas unbound cells are not. The retained cells are then recovered.

4.4 Neutralization of toxic substances

Passive antibody administration can neutralize toxic substances in emergency episodes where binding to the substance and inducing its clearance or destruction is sufficient to prevent lethal injury to the body (Section 3.3).

Poisons. Toxic substances produced by venomous snakes and poisonous insects, which consist of biologically active polypeptides and other macromolecules that are lethal to humans, can be inactivated if antitoxin antibody or antibody fragments are administered soon after exposure.

Therapeutic drugs. Digoxin is prescribed for the treatment of congestive heart failure and cardiac arrhythmias. Effective treatment requires high doses of drug and risks toxic side-effects. In cases of digoxin intoxication, the drug can be neutralized successfully and cleared with anti-digoxin Fab fragments (Section 2.5.1). Similar antibody antidotes may also be useful in cases of overdose involving colchicine and tricyclic antidepressants.

Drugs of abuse. Catalytic antibodies (Section 2.9) raised against a transition-state analog of cocaine can catalyze the hydrolysis of the benzoyl ester group of the drug and so mimic the action of natural enzymes that convert the drug into fragments devoid of stimulant activity.

4.5 Immune deficiency

In healthy individuals, the immune system is generally able to protect the body against infection by the micro-organisms in the environment to which it is continually exposed. Infants with undeveloped immune function, especially those born prematurely or suffering from malnutrition, are particularly susceptible to infection (Section 4.6.1). Immune function becomes gradually impaired with increasing age and infirmity. In a number of medical situations, the capacity of the immune system to combat infection is either absent or significantly impaired.

4.5.1 Primary immunodeficiency

Primary immunodeficiency disorders are congenital in origin, may affect one or more components of the immune system and frequently manifest during infancy or childhood.

B-cell immunodeficiencies. B-cell disorders are characterized by the absence of gamma globulin, or agammaglobulinemia, a variable reduction in multiple Ig subclasses or the selective deficiency of specific isotypes, and an increased susceptibility to infection by bacteria and some other micro-organisms.

T-cell immunodeficiencies. Defects in T-cell maturation and function impair the action of the cellular arm of the immune system and increase susceptibility to micro-organisms that establish infection within cells.

Severe combined immunodeficiencies. Combined immunodeficiencies arise by the abnormal development of both B and T lymphocytes, result in a profound loss of both cellular and humoral immunity and leave patients at extreme risk of severe infection.

4.5.2 Secondary immunodeficiency

Secondary, or acquired, immunodeficiencies develop as the result of infection (Section 4.6), cancer (Section 4.7) or medical treatment of cancer and immune-mediated disorders (Section 4.8).

Infectious diseases. Micro-organisms that establish a persistent state of infection can subvert the immune response and allow opportunistic infection by other microbes to occur. A prime example is the acquired immune deficiency syndrome (AIDS) that follows infection with the human immunodeficiency virus (HIV) (Section 4.6.2).

Cancer. Patients with advanced malignancies are often immunosuppressed because normal lymphocyte production is impeded by tumor cell multiplication in the bone marrow compartment or because tumor cells and their products interfere with the normal functioning of the immune system in some other way.

Drug therapy. A period of immune insufficiency follows high-dose chemotherapy or radiotherapy treatments for cancer that destroy bone marrow cells. Drugs such as corticosteroids and cyclosporin A, which are used to control severe inflammatory disorders and transplant rejection, cause widespread suppression of the immune system.

The infectious complications of some immune deficiency states can be ameliorated by the passive administration of polyclonal Ig (Section 5.3). Preparations of Ig naturally contain a mixture of antibodies with specificity for a variety of the common pathogens encountered by the human population, and their variants, and may be enriched in antibodies that recognize a particular pathogen to which the population has been exposed recently or repeatedly. Pathogenic microbes may also be neutralized selectively by Mabs or by combinations of Mabs that recognize different viral mutants or bacterial strains.

4.6 Microbial infection

4.6.1 Viruses

A number of common pathogenic viruses cause disease in healthy individuals. Other viruses infect a large proportion of the population but do not usually manifest their serious pathogenic effects unless the immune system of an individual is weakened (Section 4.5). Other pathogenic viruses that are not generally considered life-threatening in adults may be potentially lethal in immune-compromised patients. Infants may be at particular risk because of the high chance of viral transmission from an infected mother in the perinatal period.

Rabies virus. The rabies virus occurs in a range of wild animals and is chiefly transmitted to humans through bites from rabid dogs. Rabies virus is neurotropic and causes an acute condition called hydrophobia that is characterized by spasms, paralysis and almost inevitable death.

Cytomegalovirus. Cytomegalovirus (CMV) usually causes mild reactions in healthy individuals because it is maintained in a dormant state by the immune system. In patients with weakened immune systems, CMV can develop into a severe, life-threatening disease associated with GI tract ulcers, retinitis leading to blindness, and interstitial pneumonia.

Hepatitis B virus. Infection with hepatitis B virus (HBV) is usually mild in immune-competent individuals. Loss of tolerance to viral persistence results in hepatic inflammation, and the damage to liver cells that follows can ultimately necessitate liver transplantation. Anti-HBV antibody may be able to reduce viral load and prevent post-transplant reinfection of the donor liver.

Respiratory syncytial virus. The respiratory syncytial virus (RSV) primarily infects young children, the aged and immune-compromised patients, leading to episodes of bronchiolitis and pneumonia. RSV infection causes epidemics in pediatric hospital wards and can be fatal in children with congenital heart disease, pulmonary disorders or poor immune status.

Herpes simplex viruses. The herpes simplex viruses (HSV) are responsible for cold sores and genital warts and are associated with high mortality and permanent neurological damage in infants acquiring the infection from an affected mother.

Varicella zoster virus. The virus that is responsible for causing chicken-pox in children, varicella zoster virus (VZV), can lead to a life-threatening pneumonitis in infants who are immune-compromised. VZV also causes shingles in adults and can be life-threatening in immune-compromised individuals.

Polyclonal Ig preparations and Mabs that recognize viral surface anti-gens can block their function (Section 3.3.1), neutralize infective virus particles and limit viral spread within the body. However, such anti-bodies can have little or no effect on a virus once it has gained entry to a target cell. Thus, anti-viral antibodies are most likely to be effective when administered prophylactically to patients who are known or pre-sumed to be at risk of developing viral disease, or when given before serious infection has become established (Section 5.4.1).

4.6.2 Human immunodeficiency virus

AIDS is transmitted between individuals predominantly by exposure to blood or blood products contaminated with HIV. After initial infection with HIV, a burst of viral replication occurs within CD4 +ve T lympho-cytes (Section 1.4.3) leading to dissemination of virus throughout the body. The immune system mounts a cellular and humoral response that gives the appearance of being effective in controlling the infection. During this stage of infection, which may last for several years, symp-toms are few or absent and the virus appears to be latent in peripheral blood cells. However, viral replication actually persists throughout this time, especially within lymph nodes, leading to continuous rounds of T-cell infection, destruction and replacement. The next stage, known as the AIDS-related complex, is characterized by increasing viremia and decreasing levels of CD4 +ve T-cells, accompanied by symptoms such as fever, weight loss and diarrhea. AIDS represents the end-stage disease of HIV infection. Immunosuppression is accompanied by life-threatening opportunistic viral and bacterial infections, malignancy and dementia. The progression from infection with HIV to AIDS is thought to be influenced by a host of genetic and environmental factors. The immuno-pathology of HIV infection has proved to be complex and remains to be fully elucidated.

HIV is a retrovirus that reproduces predominantly within human CD4 +ve T lymphocytes and monocytes (*Figure 4.1*). The virus consists of two identical strands of RNA packaged within a core of viral proteins that is enveloped by a phospholipid bilayer derived from the host cell membrane. The viral envelope protein is a complex of gp120, exposed on the surface of the virion, bound noncovalently to gp41, which is embedded within the membrane. HIV associates with T cells and mononuclear phagocytes by means of a specific interaction between

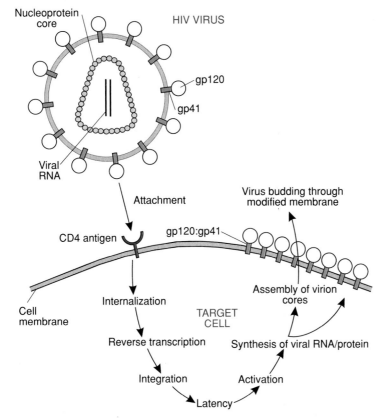

Figure 4.1: Human immunodeficiency virus and the infection of CD4 +ve cells.

gp120 and the CD4 molecule on the cell surface. Following entry of the virus into the cell, the RNA genome is transcribed into double-stranded DNA that becomes integrated into the host genome where it can remain in a latent state. T-cell activation stimulates the integrated provirus into action. Viral RNA is packaged into nucleoprotein cores in the cytoplasm. The envelope proteins are synthesized as a gp160 transmembrane precursor that becomes cleaved on the cell surface to give the gp120:gp41 complex. Virion cores that bud from the cell surface become enveloped in cell membrane bearing gp120:gp41 to yield new infective viral particles.

The principal targets of antibody therapy in AIDS are the HIV virus itself and virally infected cells. One approach is to block the interaction between the virus envelope protein gp120 and the CD4 antigen to prevent HIV entry into susceptible cells. In principle, this can be achieved using anti-gp120 antibodies (Section 3.3.1) or CD4 immunoadhesins (Section 3.3.2) that can bind to a conserved site of the viral coat protein, block the binding site for CD4, and enhance Fc receptor-mediated phagocytosis of the virus (Section 1.6.2). An alternative strategy is to target the gp120 and gp41 molecules that become expressed selectively on the surface of HIV-infected cells with immunotoxins (Section 3.6.3). The approach aims to destroy cells in which viral replication is occurring before release of further infective virus particles can occur.

Antibody treatment is most likely to be effective when used early in HIV infection before significant viral dissemination has occurred. This may be possible when the timing of infection is known, as in the case of accidental needle-stick injuries with contaminated blood. Individuals known to be at high risk of infection could be treated prophylactically. For example, treatment of HIV-infected mothers with antibody may reduce the chance of viral transmission to their offspring during birth. In later stages of infection, repeated rounds of antibody treatment would be required to both neutralize HIV and kill virus-producing cells. Antibody can have only minimal effect on latent infection or the spread of virus by cell-to-cell contact and thus is unlikely to be capable of preventing the progression to AIDS unless used as an adjunct to antiviral drugs that block viral replication extensively.

4.6.3 Gram-negative bacteria

Infection with Gram-negative bacteria is a major cause of death in intensive care units and the mortality among patients who develop bacterial sepsis is high. The gradual emergence of acquired resistance to multiple antibiotics has emphasized the need for alternative therapeutic agents such as antibodies that react with components of the bacterial outer membrane or capsule. Organisms frequently involved in causing bacterial sepsis include *Pseudomonas aeruginosa*, *Escherichia coli*, *Klebsiella pneumoniae*, *Staphylococcus aureus* and *Staphylococcus epidermidis*.

Bacteria proliferating within the body release soluble protein toxins, known as exotoxins, into the bloodstream. The membrane-derived endotoxins of Gram-negative bacteria are lipopolysaccharides that consist of three antigenic domains: O-polysaccharide, core polysaccharide and lipid A. The O-polysaccharide consists of multiple repeating oligosaccharide units and defines different bacterial species and serotypes. The core oligosaccharide is highly conserved within a given bacterial species and some regions of structure are conserved across species. The lipid A structure is highly conserved across bacterial strains and species and is the component responsible for the biological effects of endotoxins.

The mechanism by which endotoxin gives rise to toxic effects involves the binding of lipid A to a serum glycoprotein, the lipopolysaccharide-binding protein, to form a complex that interacts with the monocyte-macrophage cell surface antigen CD14. Activated macrophages release a variety of inflammatory mediators of which TNF-α is an early and key component. TNF-α stimulates other macrophages to secrete IL-1, IL-6, IL-8, platelet-activating factor (PAF), prostaglandin D_2, leukotrienes and more TNF-α. In combination with the other cytokines, TNF-α activates neutrophils and endothelial cells and promotes a systemic inflammatory response syndrome (SIRS) called septic shock (Section 4.8.3).

For effective therapy or prophylaxis, anti-bacterial antibodies should bind with the key serotypes involved in major infections. Recognition of multiple serotypes can be achieved either by using broadly reactive polyclonal Ig or by using combinations, or cocktails, of Mabs that react with antigenic polysaccharide structures of different serotype. The bacterial endotoxins that trigger macrophage activation are believed to be key mediators in the induction of the inflammatory cascade. Mabs inactivating the common lipid A antigen could prevent or hinder the development of septic shock in the face of severe infection with Gram-negative bacteria. An alternative approach would be to block the lipopolysaccharide-binding protein. The prominent role of TNF-α in inflammation suggests that either anti-TNF-α Mabs (Section 3.3.1) or TNF receptor immunoadhesins (Section 3.3.2) could potentially block the inflammatory cascade at an early stage, although other mediators released by activated macrophages contribute to the development of the shock syndrome (Section 5.4.2).

4.6.4 Enteric infections

A number of viral, bacterial and parasitic infections of the GI tract could potentially be countered by the enteric administration of antibody preparations capable of preventing the attachment of microbes to the gut epithelial cells within which they replicate (Section 2.2). Species of *Shigella* are responsible for traveler's diarrhea. *Cryptosporidium parvum* is a parasite that causes diarrhea in healthy individuals but can spread from the intestine to internal organs in immune deficient patients to cause death. *Rotavirus* infection is associated with diarrhea, fever and vomiting leading to dehydration that can be fatal in infants. *Helicobacter pylori* is thought to be responsible for the formation and recurrence of gastric ulcers and has been implicated in cancers of the stomach. A complication with the use of broad-spectrum antibiotics is that elimination of the native bacterial flora of the GI tract allows opportunistic infection by disease-causing organisms such as *Clostridium difficile* that would not normally colonize the gut successfully.

4.6.5 Pseudomonas *infection in cystic fibrosis*

Pseudomonas aeruginosa frequently infects the lungs of patients with cystic fibrosis. The basic molecular defect underlying the clinical manifestation of cystic fibrosis is mutation in a transmembrane conductance regulator that controls chloride ion permeability at the luminal epithelial surface. Abnormal ion transport reduces the water content in the airway, giving rise to thickened intraluminal secretions that facilitate the establishment of bacterial infection. *Pseudomonas* infection attracts inflammatory cells that contribute to further thickening of the mucus in the lung. A mucoid exopolysaccharide that protects the bacterium against destruction by leukocytes may serve as a target for antibody therapy.

4.7 Cancer

The survival and multiplication of cells in the body is tightly controlled to ensure that the behavior of each cell type is appropriate to its location and function in the body. Genetic mutation can subvert the normal responses of cells to growth regulatory mechanisms (see Sections 4.7.3 and 4.7.4). The inappropriate proliferation of such abnormal cells gives rise to tumors. The phenotype of tumor cells varies according to the tissue of origin, the oncogenic mutations involved, and the natural history of the tumor's development. Tumors are generally classified by their cell or tissue of origin, their cellular appearance and their behavior (*Table 4.3*).

Cancers growing as discrete lumps are commonly referred to as solid tumors (Section 4.7.6). Benign tumors are localized and do not spread away from the site of origin. Surgery and localized radiotherapy are

Table 4.3: Common malignant tumor types treated by antibody therapy

Tissue of origin	Tumor type	Cell of origin
Breast	Adenocarcinoma	Epithelial cell
Colon, rectum	Adenocarcinoma	Epithelial cell
Lung	Adenocarcinoma Small cell carcinoma	Epithelial cell Neuroendocrine cell
Ovary	Adenocarcinoma	Epithelial cell
Head, neck	Squamous cell carcinoma	Epithelial cell
Liver	Hepatoma	Epithelial cell
Skin	Malignant melanoma	Pigment cell
Nervous system	Neuroblastoma Glioblastoma	Nerve cell Glial cell
Blood	Leukemia	Monocytes Granulocytes Lymphocytes
Lymph node	Non-Hodgkin's lymphoma Hodgkin's lymphoma	Lymphocyte Reticuloendothelial cell

common treatments for such tumors. In contrast, malignant tumors are characterized by invasion of surrounding tissues, entry to lymphatic tissues and blood, and establishment at secondary sites, or metastases (Section 4.7.7), distant from the site of origin. In this case, systemic therapy with chemotherapeutic drugs or radiation is necessary because local treatment of the primary tumor alone is insufficient once metastasis has occurred. Tumors of the hematopoietic system (Section 1.4.1), called leukemias, spread throughout the bone marrow and blood and may form discrete masses in lymph nodes and other organs. Lymphomas originate from lymph node cells and spread into the blood and other tissues. Both leukemias and lymphomas require systemic therapy because tumor cells become distributed throughout the body.

Current systemic treatments fail when they cannot eradicate tumor at the maximum doses of chemotherapy or radiotherapy compatible with tolerable toxic side-effects on normal tissues, especially proliferating tissues such as the stem cells of the bone marrow and the epithelium of the GI tract. The aim of antibody therapy of cancer is to substitute or supplement conventional modes of treatment by directly targeting tumor cells or by triggering anti-tumor immune effects selectively so as to minimize side-effects on nonmalignant cells (Section 5.5).

4.7.1 Tumor-associated antigens

Tumor cells can be distinguished from their normal counterparts by the pattern of antigenic molecules that they express. A tumor-associated antigen (TAA) reflects both the origin and the phenotypic properties of a particular tumor type. Accordingly, different tumor types exhibit characteristic TAAs on their cell surfaces (*Table 4.4*). In many cases, the antigens strongly associated with the tumor are simply differentiation antigens that reflect the cell of origin. In other cases, a normal cell surface component such as a growth factor receptor, which is usually expressed only at low levels on the tissue of origin, is expressed at elevated levels by the tumor cell. A third category of antigen is represented by so-called oncofetal antigens that are usually expressed by undifferentiated cells during development and not by differentiated cells. Fourthly, cancer cells frequently have altered patterns of glycosylation so that new epitopes are formed and peptide determinants are revealed that are largely concealed on normal cells.

The value of a particular TAA for antibody therapy is related to its distribution on tumor versus normal tissues. TAAs are rarely restricted to tumor cells alone and are generally also present on a number of normal tissues. The expression of a target antigen on nonvital tissues or on cells that can be replaced by the body does not preclude therapy provided that access of antibody to the tumor itself is not significantly impeded by adsorption to antigen not associated with the tumor. In

Table 4.4: Tumor-associated antigens as targets of antibody therapy

Tumor type	Tumor-associated antigen	Properties
Carcinomas	Polymorphic epithelial mucin (PEM)	>100 kDa Glycoprotein
	Epithelial membrane antigen (EMA)	40 kDa Glycoprotein
	Carcinoembryonic antigen (CEA)	180 kDa Glycoprotein
	Glycoprotein-72 (gp72)	72 kDa Glycoprotein
	Epidermal growth factor (EGF) receptor	175 kDa Glycoprotein
	c-*erb*B2/HER-2 receptor	185 kDa Glycoprotein
Hepatoma	Ferritin	Secreted protein
Malignant melanoma	High molecular weight melanoma-associated antigen (HMW-MAA)	>450 kDa Chondroitin sulfate glycoprotein
	GD2	Ganglioside
	GD3	Ganglioside
Neuroendocrine tumors	Neural cell adhesion molecules (CD56)	180 kDa Glycoprotein
	GD2	Ganglioside
Glioblastoma	Tenascin	Extracellular matrix protein
Myeloid leukemia	CD33	67 kDa Glycoprotein
T-cell leukemia	IL-2 receptor α chain (CD25)	55 kDa Protein
	CAMPATH antigen (CD52)	20 kDa Glycoprotein
B-cell tumors	Idiotype	Surface Ig
	CD19	90 kDa Glycoprotein
	CD20	35 kDa Protein
	CD22	135/140 kDa Glycoproteins
	CD37	40–52 kDa Glycoproteins
Hodgkin's lymphoma	CD30	105–120 kDa Glycoprotein

some circumstances, the presence of a target antigen on vital normal tissues is not an obstacle to therapy because the tissue resides in a part of the body that is not readily accessible to administered antibody. The degree of expression of TAAs on tumors can vary between tumors in different patients, between tumors at different sites within the same patient, and between tumor cells at the same site. Antigenic heterogeneity can be addressed by using cocktails of Mabs that recognize different target antigens on the same tumor type, although the risk of cross-reactivity with normal tissue is thereby increased and so the selectivity of tumor targeting may be reduced. Alternatively, therapies that are capable of exerting effects on bystander cells, such as immune stimulation (Section 3.4), RAIT (Sections 3.6.1 and 3.7.1) and ADEPT (Section 3.7.2), can eliminate target antigen-negative cells in the vicinity of targeted tumor cells.

The properties of a TAA influence the choice of the optimal strategy for antibody therapy. The density of antigen on the surface of a target cell dictates the maximum amount of antibody or immunoconjugate that can bind and hence the magnitude of the therapeutic effect. Certain antigens persist on the cell membrane and are good targets for approaches that require action at the cell surface, such as immune stimulation (Section 3.4) and two-stage targeting (Section 3.7). Antigenic modulation may lead to the internalization of some antigens when cross-linked by antibody, thus removing Mab or immunoconjugate from the cell surface (Section 1.6.1). Other antigens become internalized by cells via routes that promote the action of antibody-targeted agents such as radionuclides, chemotherapeutic drugs and toxins (Section 3.6). Antigens may also be shed from the tumor cell surface into the circulation and so hinder the binding of Mab to the cell-associated target antigen (Section 5.5.1).

4.7.2 B-cell idiotypes

Non-Hodgkin's lymphoma and chronic lymphocytic leukemia arise from cells of the B lymphocyte lineage and generally display Ig molecules on the cell surface (Section 1.4.2). The monoclonal origin of such tumors means that every cancer cell expresses the same V regions and hence the same idiotype (Section 1.3.7). Moreover, certain idiotopes of the surface Ig, the 'private' determinants, represent truly unique antigenic targets. For practical purposes, Mabs directed against the idiotype of the surface Ig on a B-cell tumor can be considered almost entirely tumor-specific. A limitation of the B-cell idiotype as a target is that every patient's tumor is unique and so treatment requires that an individualized anti-id Mab be raised in each case (Section 5.5.1). An alternative approach is to develop panels of Mabs that recognize shared or 'semi-public' idiotypic determinants and can therefore cross-react with tumors from multiple patients. However, components of Mab panels also cross-react more extensively with normal B lymphocytes.

The surface Ig of a B-cell tumor may be used as a 'personal' vaccine to stimulate an immune response to the patient's unique idiotype The procedure generally involves the immortalization of lymphoma cells from patient biopsies to provide a source of Ig for vaccination (*Figure 4.2*). The advantage of the approach is that vaccination can generate a polyclonal immune response recognizing multiple idiotypic determinants and so make escape mutants less likely to emerge (Section 5.5.1). However, the routine preparation of patient-specific Ig by this means is not straightforward. A novel approach employs PCR to amplify the V_H and V_L domain gene sequences from a patient's lymphoma cells (*Figure 4.2*). The cloned V domain genes can be manipulated to express recombinant antibody scFv fragments (Section 2.5.2) that bear the idiotype of the surface Ig. The procedure may simplify and accelerate the production of specific Ig for individualized vaccines. An alternative approach to

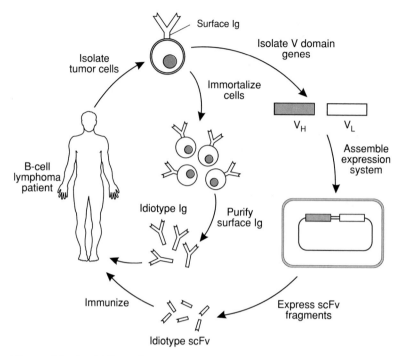

Figure 4.2: Anti-idiotypic vaccination.

vaccination involves the direct injection of DNA gene vectors carrying V domain genes into muscle to express the antibody fragment *in vivo*.

4.7.3 Growth factors and receptors

Cell growth is regulated by a balance between stimulatory and inhibitory signals transmitted to a cell by means of receptors that detect contact with neighboring cells or stroma and receptors that bind to soluble growth regulatory factors (*Figure 4.3*). A tumor cell can enhance its rate of division by increasing the output of a growth factor that stimulates receptors on its surface, a phenomenon known as autocrine stimulation. Alternatively, in paracrine stimulation, a tumor cell that expresses an elevated level of a growth factor receptor can be more readily stimulated by growth factors produced by another tumor or normal cell. Growth factors such as IL-2 and EGF and their receptors have been implicated in the regulation of a number of tumor types (*Table 4.4*).

Antibody neutralization of growth factors can halt tumor proliferation but requires the continuous presence of the antibody and leaves the tumor intact. An alternative approach is to target growth factor receptors that are expressed on the tumor cell surface. Many growth factor receptors are transmembrane glycoproteins comprising an extracellular

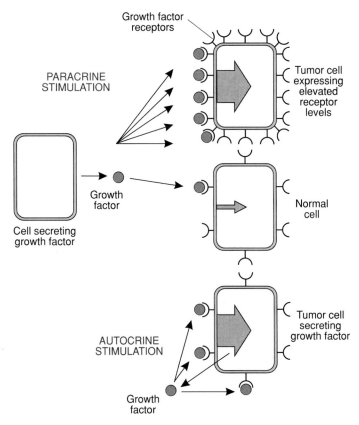

Figure 4.3: Growth factor stimulation of tumor cells.

domain that binds the soluble factor and an intracellular domain involved in signal transduction. Mabs that bind to the extracellular portions of a growth factor receptor can block the binding site of the receptor directly and so prevent interaction with its ligand (Section 3.3.1). Alternatively, Mabs can cause growth factor receptors to become down-regulated from the cell surface so that they can no longer function. In some instances, Mab agonists binding to nonblocking epitopes of a surface receptor can transduce signals that reduce cell viability or increase sensitivity to chemotherapeutic agents.

4.7.4 Apoptosis

Apoptosis is a natural form of programed cell death characterized by membrane blebbing, condensation of cytoplasm, segmentation of the nucleus, aggregation of chromatin and endonucleolytic fragmentation of genomic DNA. Apoptosis is quite distinct from necrosis, the cellular disintegration that occurs as the pathological consequence of unnatural physical or chemical damage. Genetic mutation affecting the apoptotic mechanisms that control cell number in tissues can lead to the uncontrolled multiplication of cells. Mabs that bind to the APO-1 or Fas antigen, a transmembrane glycoprotein present on human B and T lymphocytes, can induce the apoptotic death of leukemic cells in tissue culture and in animal models. Cross-linking of APO-1 molecules at the cell surface by a Mab agonist transduces a cytolytic signal into the cell without the need for activation of accessory immune effector mechanisms. Another approach is to use a Mab to target inhibitors of cell signaling enzymes, such as the naturally occurring drug genistein, that can interfere with the function of target antigen receptor-associated tyrosine kinases and induce apoptotic cell death.

4.7.5 Angiogenesis

Normal tissues are perfused by a vascular network that supplies oxygen and essential nutrients. The growth of tumors that arise *in situ* is limited by the ability of nutrients to diffuse into the tumor mass from surrounding tissues and blood vessels. The transition from an *in situ* tumor to an invasive carcinoma is dependent upon the formation of new blood vessels. Ordinarily, this process, called neovascularization or angiogenesis, is tightly controlled and occurs only during development, reproduction and wound healing. Tumors, however, produce specific angiogenic factors, such as basic fibroblast growth factor (bFGF) and vascular endothelial growth factor (VEGF), that promote the migration and proliferation of endothelial cells from existing vessels to form new tumor vasculature (*Figure 4.4*). Mabs interfering with the action of bFGF and VEGF or their cellular receptors (Section 3.3.1) may block the enlargement of solid tumors by inhibiting further vascularization. The expression of the integrin $\alpha_V\beta_3$ (CD51/CD61), also known as the vitronectin receptor, on vascular endothelial cells responding to angiogenic stimuli appears necessary both for their survival and for their ultimate differentiation. Mab antagonists that block $\alpha_V\beta_3$ can inhibit the growth of human tumors by selectively promoting apoptosis of the proliferating neovascular cells while leaving pre-existing quiescent blood vessels unaffected.

4.7.6 Solid tumors

The cellular architecture of solid tumors (*Figure 4.5*) limits the efficacy of antibody therapy. The peripheral rim of a solid cancer tends to be well vascularized and to contain rapidly dividing tumor cells. In contrast, the avascular center of a solid tumor is necrotic and contains dead or degenerating cells. The perfusion of solid cellular masses is heterogeneous. Blood flow to certain regions of the tumor is poor because the

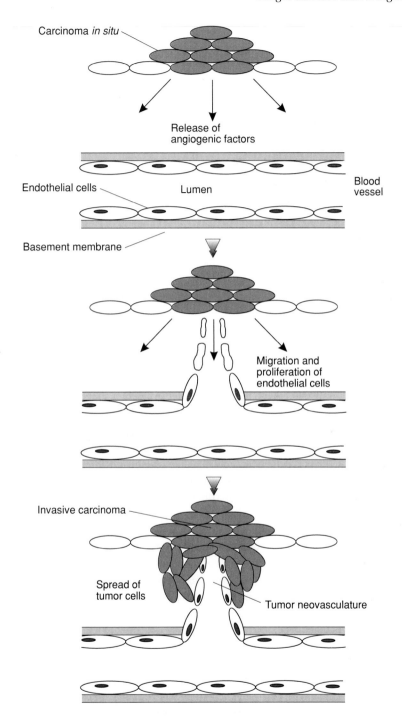

Figure 4.4: Steps in the development of invasive carcinoma.

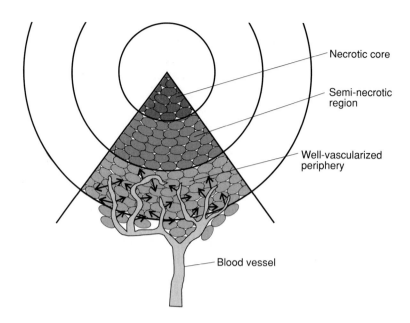

Figure 4.5: The cellular architecture of solid tumors.

neovasculature is disorganized. It may be possible to increase blood flow by local irradiation or by targeting vasoactive agents with antibody (Section 3.9.1). Solid tumors have no lymphatic drainage, causing a high interstitial pressure in the tumor core that counters the movement of large molecules such as antibodies which are predominantly transported by convection. The use of smaller antibody fragments with better diffusion characteristics can improve the degree of tumor penetration (Section 2.5).

The penetration of antibody to the core of a solid tumor mass is limited by initial adsorption to cells at the tumor periphery. Healthy tumor cells that express target antigen are present directly adjacent to blood vessels and can act as a sink for antibody entering the tumor. The amount of antibody available to move into the core of a tumor is thereby decreased, allowing tumor cells in the semi-necrotic region to escape treatment. The localization of antibody in the periphery of the tumor may prove effective when used to deliver agents that can potentially penetrate to the center of the tumor, as in RAIT (Sections 3.6.1 and 3.7.1) and ADEPT (Section 3.7.2). An alternative approach, called tumor necrosis therapy, seeks to target antigens that are present in the center of a tumor but are absent from its periphery and so do not hinder penetration by antibody. Necrotic cells are permeable and allow leakage of cellular components such as nuclear proteins that are not normally released from healthy tissues.

4.7.7 Metastasis

Metastasis, the spread of cancer from its site of origin, is a multi-step process (*Figure 4.6*). In the first step, tumor cells invade and infiltrate surrounding normal tissues. The tumor cells adhere less tightly to normal tissue and produce hydrolytic enzymes that destroy the connective tissue between cells and organs. Individual cells, or clumps of cells, within the tumor mass then enter the lymph or blood. A proportion may survive to travel in the bloodstream to other tissues and organs and become entrapped in capillary beds. Penetration into surrounding tissue involves adhesion to endothelial cells and the action of enzymes that can degrade basement membrane. Tumor cells are known to express cell surface molecules that endow them with enhanced metastatic properties. A variant form of the CD44 antigen, an adhesion molecule that binds hyaluronate and is transiently expressed on lymphocytes present within lymph nodes, is associated with more highly metastatic tumor cells. Mabs that block such adhesion molecules can inhibit the process of metastatis.

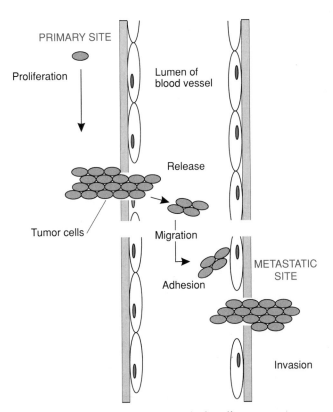

Figure 4.6: The metastatic spread of malignant tumor.

4.7.8 Multidrug resistance

A major reason for the failure of chemotherapy to eradicate tumor cells completely is the development of resistance by malignant cells to multiple cytotoxic agents. The multidrug resistance phenotype is commonly characterized by overproduction of a membrane protein, known as gp170 or P-glycoprotein, which is a transmembrane pump that drives the expulsion of chemotherapeutic drugs from the interior of the cell. Mabs that bind to certain epitopes on the extracellular domain of P-glycoprotein can block its function, inhibit drug efflux and thereby increase the sensitivity of target cells to chemotherapeutic drugs.

4.8 Immune-mediated disorders

4.8.1 Inflammation

The inflammatory response is the body's protective reaction to the presence of foreign material, infection or injury (Sections 4.8.2 and 4.8.3). Inflammation is also associated with a number of common immune-mediated disorders, including autoimmune diseases (Section 4.8.4), transplant rejection (Section 4.8.5) and allergy (Section 4.8.6). The response is characterized by dilation of the blood capillaries at the site of insult, increased blood flow to the site, influx of plasma and migration of leukocytes across the vessel wall into the tissue. The recruitment of leukocytes in inflammation is a complex multi-step process (*Figure 4.7*) in which cell adhesion molecules present on the surface of both leukocytes and endothelial cells play a prominent role (*Table 4.5*).

Infection or damage to tissue stimulates resident macrophages to release chemical signals that activate endothelial cells lining nearby blood vessels. Endothelial cells respond by increasing expression of P-selectin rapidly and the levels of E-selectin increase subsequently in response to the pro-inflammatory cytokines TNF-α and IL-1. The selectins mediate the initial attachment of leukocytes to the vessel wall. Leukocytes traveling in the flowing bloodstream make contact with the endothelium and their movement is slowed to a rolling motion. The relatively weak and reversible tethering allows the leukocytes to become exposed to key activating signals. Chemoattractant factors such as N-formylated peptides, complement C5a fragment, leukotriene B_4, PAF and chemokines such as IL-8 and monocyte chemotactic protein-1, trigger activation of the integrins LFA-1, Mac-1 and VLA-4. The movement of the leukocytes along the endothelium is arrested by tighter binding between the integrins and Ig superfamily receptors on the surface of the endothelium. The receptor ICAM-1 predominates on activated endothelial cells responding to TNF-α, IL-1 and IFN-γ. The expression of VCAM-1 is triggered by TNF-α, IL-1 and also IL-4. The

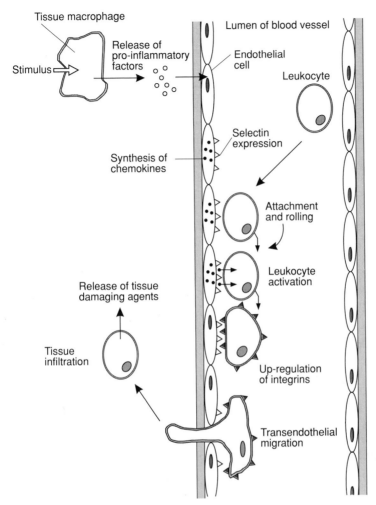

Figure 4.7: Steps in the mechanism of leukocyte-mediated inflammation.

strongly adhering leukocytes then change their morphology and migrate across the blood vessel wall to the site of injury.

Antibody therapy has the potential to intervene at several steps in the process of leukocyte recruitment. Mabs may neutralize the pro-inflammatory complement peptides, cytokines and chemokines that attract leukocytes and stimulate the expression of adhesion molecules on both leukocytes and endothelium (Section 3.3.1). Alternatively, Mabs that bind selectively to adhesion molecules can block both the weak selectin-mediated interactions that occur early in the inflammation process and the later strong integrin-mediated interactions between adherent cells.

Table 4.5: Cellular adhesion molecules involved in inflammation

Molecule	Expressing cells	Binding cells	Ligand
Selectins			
P-selectin (CD62P)	Activated endothelium Platelets Megakaryocytes	Monocytes Neutrophils Platelets	Sialylated fucosylated molecules
E-selectin (CD62E)	Activated endothelium	Monocytes Neutrophils Eosinophils Basophils	
L-selectin (CD62L)	Lymphocytes Monocytes Neutrophils	Activated endothelium High endothelial venules	GlyCAM-1 MadCAM-1 CD34
Integrins			
LFA-1 (CD18/CD11a)	Monocytes Lymphocytes Neutrophils	Endothelial cells Monocytes Lymphocytes	ICAM-1 (CD54) ICAM-2 (CD102)
Mac-1 (CD18/CD11b)	Monocytes Neutrophils NK cells	Endothelial cells Monocytes Lymphocytes	ICAM-1 (CD54)
VLA-4 (CD29/CD49d)	Thymocytes Lymphocytes Eosinophils	Endothelial cells Macrophages	VCAM-1 (CD106)

4.8.2 Ischemia and reperfusion injury

Ischemia is a condition of tissue oxygen deprivation caused by a temporary blockade or a reduction in blood flow that is characteristic of a variety of clinical conditions. Localized ischemia occurs in stroke, myocardial infarction (MI) and acute renal failure and causes elevated tissue levels of pro-inflammatory mediators that up-regulate the expression of adhesion molecules on neutrophils and endothelial cells. Reperfusion, the restoration of normal blood flow, is crucial to recovery of organ function, yet is frequently associated with inflammatory damage to tissues because neutrophils attach to activated endothelium and release tissue-damaging oxygen radicals, proteases and vasoactive substances. Oxygen radicals in turn stimulate the production of chemotactic factors such as IL-8 that promote neutrophil infiltration. The result is damage to endothelial cells, loss of vascular integrity, edema, hemorrhage, obstruction of capillaries and extensive local tissue injury. Intervention with Mabs targeting key steps in the inflammatory cascade may control the damaging response to reperfusion of ischemic tissue (Section 4.8.1).

4.8.3 Systemic inflammatory response syndrome

Noninfectious stimuli, such as multiple trauma and severe burns, as well as severe infections with bacteria, fungi, parasites or viruses, can lead to SIRS (Section 4.6.3). As a result of the direct effects of a number of mediators released by monocytes and macrophages, neutrophils become activated, adhere to vascular endothelial cells and penetrate to the tissues. The combination of potent mediators and activated neutrophils results in extensive damage to the vasculature and causes refractory hypotension. Other events that can be triggered include activation of the complement pathway, the coagulation cascade and the generation of bradykinin. The consequences of uncontrolled systemic inflammation include myocardial dysfunction, acute renal failure, acute respiratory distress, hepatic failure and disseminated intravascular coagulation, followed by complete failure of vital organ systems. Mabs blocking the cell surface antigens involved in the activation and action of neutrophils may be able to mitigate the consequences of systemic release of pro-inflammatory mediators (Section 4.8.1).

4.8.4 Autoimmune disease

Autoimmune diseases are characterized by the reaction of the body's immune system with self antigens (*Table 4.6*). In some disorders, e.g. myasthenia gravis, autoantibodies interfere with the function of a cell-associated self antigen within a particular organ. In other cases, e.g. systemic lupus erythematosus, autoantibodies form immune complexes with a circulating self antigen, deposit in blood vessels in various organs and cause vasculitis, or vascular inflammation. In a number of other diseases, notably rheumatoid arthritis and multiple sclerosis, cytopathic effects are mediated by lymphocytes and macrophages. A common feature of several autoimmune disorders is a chronic inflammatory state that tends to follow an irregular pattern of remission and relapse.

T lymphocytes can become activated when self-tolerance mechanisms (Section 1.4.5) fail or are overridden, a situation that may occur as a result of certain infections. A prominent feature of many autoimmune diseases is the presence of activated CD4 +ve helper T cells (Section 1.4.3) that are key to the induction and maintenance of inflammation. The event that triggers an autoimmune response involves specific activation of autoreactive T-cell subsets by antigen-presenting cells (APCs) bearing self-antigen peptides in association with MHC class II molecules (*Figure 4.8*). In the next phase, the activated T cells release cytokines and activate other immune cells (Section 1.4.3). IL-2 stimulates the autocrine and paracrine proliferation of antigen-activated T-cells. IFN-γ activates macrophages and up-regulates MHC class II expression on macrophages and other cell types. TNF-α stimulates macrophages to

Table 4.6: Characteristics of autoimmune diseases

Disease	Site	Autoantibody	Mechanism	Symptoms
Systemic lupus erythematosus	Systemic	DNA Nucleoprotein	Immune complex deposition	Inflammation of skin and kidney
Myasthenia gravis	Nerve and muscle	Acetylcholine receptor Synapse proteins	Blockade and down-regulation of receptor	Progressive muscle weakening
Multiple sclerosis	Brain and spinal cord	Myelin basic protein Oligodendroglial proteins	Destruction of myelin and nerve fibers	Visual impairment, spasticity and paralysis
Rheumatoid arthritis	Joints	Type II collagen Connective tissue	Joint inflammation and destruction of cartilage	Pain and swelling of synovial joints
Diabetes mellitus type I (juvenile onset)	Pancreas	Insulin Islet cell proteins	Destruction of beta cells of pancreatic islets	Insulin-dependent diabetes
Inflammatory bowel disease	Gastrointestinal tract	Colonic antigens	Inflammation of intestinal wall	Abdominal pain, diarrhea and bleeding

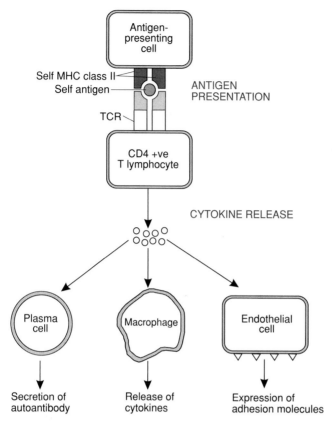

Figure 4.8: Mechanism of chronic inflammation in autoimmune disease.

release other cytokines, including IL-1, IL-6, IL-8 and more of both TNF-α and IFN-γ, and up-regulates the expression of adhesion molecules present on leukocytes and endothelial cells (Section 4.8.1). The final step involves the action of immune effector mechanisms. Macrophages release cytokines, oxygen radicals and hydrolytic enzymes that damage tissues directly. B lymphocytes produce autoantibodies that may contribute to the inflammatory process by complement activation. The chronic and cyclical nature of autoimmune diseases suggests that periodic reactivation of autoreactive T cells occurs because of repeated self-antigen presentation.

A major goal in antibody therapy of autoimmune disease is to prevent the induction of T-cell activation or to re-establish a state of tolerance to self antigen by modulating the function of T cells. Mabs that recognize T-cell antigens such as CD4 or CD52 selectively target T cells for destruction or elimination (Section 5.7.3). Nonlytic antibodies against certain T-cell antigens, in particular CD4 Mabs, are capable of inducing long-term tolerance in experimental models. A second strategy aims to interfere with the process of T-cell activation. Mabs binding to the

Table 4.7: Antigens involved in T-cell recognition and activation

T lymphocyte	Antigen-presenting cell
MHC recognition	
T-cell receptor	MHC: peptide complex
CD3	
CD4	MHC class II
CD8	MHC class I
Co-stimulation	
CD2	LFA-3 (CD58)
CD28	B7-1
CTLA-4	B7-2
LFA-1	ICAM-1
	ICAM-2

invariant regions of the TCR and MHC class II molecules can block the process of self-antigen presentation. The approach can be made more selective by targeting the MHC class II types and TCR subfamilies that are most strongly associated with particular autoimmune disorders. However, autoimmune disease generally involves multiple self-antigens and oligoclonal T-cell responses in an individual, and several MHC class II types in the susceptible population. The process of T-cell activation by APCs can also be inhibited by blocking cell-surface molecules that promote adhesion or transmit co-stimulatory signals between the two cell types (*Table 4.7*).

Inflammatory reactions that have already been triggered by T-cell activation may be interrupted by using Mabs to block the action of pro-inflammatory cytokines, especially TNF-α (Section 5.7.2), and the cellular adhesion molecules involved in leukocyte recruitment (Section 4.8.1).

4.8.5 Transplant rejection

The transplantation of cells, tissues or organs from one individual to a second individual is undertaken to ameliorate a number of serious and life-threatening conditions. Transplants usually take place between a donor and a recipient who have different genetic backgrounds, in partic-ular, with mismatched MHC antigens, and are consequently known as allografts. A major problem with allotransplantation is the risk of graft rejection that exists because the recipient's immune system can recog-nize the donor graft as foreign (Section 1.4.3). Organ allograft rejection may occur by a number of processes. In hyperacute rejection, which occurs within days of grafting, pre-existing antibodies in the recipient bind to the donor organ endothelium, activate complement and cause rapid thrombotic occlusion of blood vessels. Rapid rejection can be min-

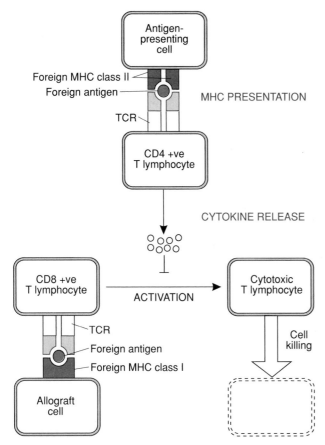

Figure 4.9: Mechanism of acute allograft rejection.

imized by close matching of donor and recipient for major blood group and MHC antigens. Acute rejection occurs within a few months of transplantation and is characterized by cellular necrosis. This form of rejection is mediated by the cellular arm of the immune response and involves the recruitment and activation of T lymphocytes. Chronic rejection, characterized by extensive fibrotic and ischemic damage to organs, may occur in the longer term, although the underlying mechanisms are not well understood.

The mechanism of the acute rejection reaction involves several components of the immune system (*Figure 4.9*). Mismatched organ transplants bear foreign MHC class I and class II molecules in association with foreign antigens, or alloantigens, and present a strong stimulus to the recipient's immune system. CD4 +ve T cells of the recipient are stimulated by the allogeneic class II MHC molecules presented by APCs in the graft. These APCs may be so-called 'passenger' leukocytes that are carried along in the graft inadvertently. The activated CD4 +ve T cells can stimulate antibody production and activate macrophages and other leukocytes by cytokine release (Section 4.8.4). CD8 +ve T cells of the recipient also become stimulated by the allogeneic MHC class I molecules expressed on endothelial and parenchymal cells of the graft. The activated CD4 +ve T cells provide the co-stimulatory cytokine signals that trigger the proliferation and differentiation of alloreactive CD8 +ve T cells. The mature alloreactive cytotoxic T lymphocytes then attack the graft tissue directly.

Antibodies have the potential to suppress the immune responses leading to acute rejection of organ transplants. Two different strategies are possible. The first is to reduce the immunogenicity of the graft itself. Donor organs may be treated *ex vivo* with Mabs that recognize passenger leukocytes within the graft. Pre-treatment of the transplant organ *ex vivo* prevents the risk that the targeting Mab will cross react with the patient's own leukocytes. Following implantation, antibody that has associated with the passenger leukocytes can activate the recipient's complement system and selectively destroy the cells before they are able to trigger T-cell activation. The second approach is to interfere directly with the action of the recipient's T lymphocytes. Polyclonal anti-thymocyte globulin (ATG) and anti-lymphocyte globulin (ALG) react broadly with T cells to cause immune suppression. Mabs recognizing T-cell-associated antigens, including the CD3 antigen, the TCR and the IL-2 receptor (Section 1.4.3), can also suppress the cellular immune responses that lead to graft rejection (Section 5.6). Both CD4 +ve and CD8 +ve T cells play an important role in acute organ rejection. Therefore, combinations of CD4 and CD8 Mabs may be necessary to establish long-term and selective tolerance to alloantigens.

4.8.6 Graft-versus-host disease

Bone marrow transplantation is undertaken in patients with disorders such as aplastic anemia, congenital enzymopathies, globin disorders, immunodeficiency and leukemias. Transplantation requires the ablation of the recipient's own bone marrow to allow the transplanted stem cells to establish and then to reconstitute the hematopoietic system. Recipients of mismatched allogeneic bone marrow transplants frequently develop the life-threatening complication of graft-versus-host disease (GVHD). In this condition, mature donor T cells carried in the marrow graft recognize the recipient's tissues as foreign. Acute GVHD is characterized by epithelial cell necrosis of skin, liver and GI tract. Chronic GVHD involves fibrosis and atrophy of organs. The incidence of GVHD can be reduced by treating the donor marrow to eliminate T cells before transplantation (Section 4.3.1). However, the efficient elimination of T cells reduces the success rate of engraftment and, in patients with certain leukemias, can lead to a higher incidence of malignant relapse. An alternative approach, which can be combined with bone marrow purging, is to target the reactive donor T cells in the recipient directly following bmt (Section 5.7.3).

4.8.7 Allergy

The allergic reaction is an excessive immune response to a common environmental antigen or a foreign substance that is normally harmless. Common allergens include grass pollen, dust mites, animal fur, certain foods, drugs and insect stings. In atopic individuals who are prone to develop strong allergic responses, and who have previously been sensitized by exposure to an allergen, a second contact with the allergen results in an immediate hypersensitivity reaction. The clinical manifestations of the response depend on whether exposure occurs through skin contact (atopic dermatitis or eczema), inhalation (allergic rhinitis and asthma), ingestion (food allergy) or injection (anaphylaxis).

Atopic individuals have high levels of circulating serum IgE and are genetically predisposed to produce large amounts of IgE in response to allergen. Initial contact with allergen is asymptomatic. At this time, antigen presentation activates allergen-specific CD4 +ve T helper cells of the T_H2 type that secrete IL-4 and induce B cells to mature into plasma cells expressing allergen-specific IgE (Section 1.4.3). IgE molecules attach to high-affinity IgE receptors (FcεRI) on mast cells that are resident in the tissues and on basophils circulating in the bloodstream (*Figure 4.10*). On a subsequent exposure, the allergen can associate immediately with and cross-link the receptor-bound IgE. The resultant dimerization of the FcεRI receptor on the cell surface transduces a signal to the mast cell that stimulates it to produce a number of key allergic mediators, including histamine, prostaglandin D_2, leukotrienes, PAF and cytokines. The acute response occurs rapidly and is characterized by increased vascular permeability, vasodilation and smooth muscle contraction.

The acute phase is followed by the development of a chronic phase characterized by a local inflammatory reaction in which activated T cells, mast cells, macrophages and infiltrating eosinophils predominate. Activated T helper cells secrete a number of cytokines. IL-4 plays a pivotal role in stimulating further production of allergen-specific IgE and induces endothelial cells to express the adhesion molecules ICAM-1 and VCAM-1 (Section 4.8.1). IL-5 plays a major role in promoting eosinophil maturation, recruitment and activation, accompanied by IL-3 and GM-CSF (Section 1.4.1). IL-10 suppresses CD4 +ve T helper cells of the T_H1 type and helps maintain the T_H2-driven allergic response. IL-3, IL-4 and IL-5 are also produced by activated mast cells and GM-CSF by macrophages and eosinophils. The activated eosinophils cause tissue damage by the release of degradative enzymes.

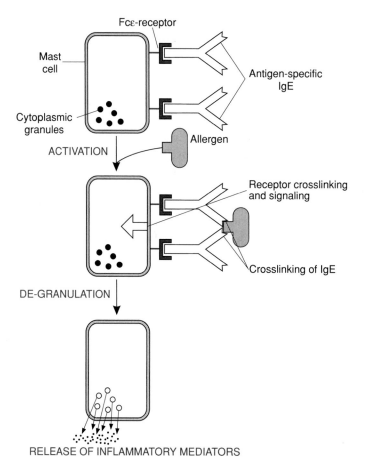

Figure 4.10: Mast cell activation by allergen.

One approach to antibody therapy of allergy is to desensitize patients in a controlled fashion by immunizing them with anti-id Mabs that mimic the antigenic structure of the allergen (Section 3.5.1). Stimulation with Mabs, rather than with the allergen, may induce the preferential development of T_H1 helper cells, leading to production of IgG rather than IgE upon repeated exposure to antigen. A second approach is to reduce or eliminate IgE itself. The approach is feasible because IgE, although known to provide a defense against certain parasitic infections, has no other apparent role in immunity. Mabs that bind selectively to regions of IgE involved in binding to FcεRI can target either circulating IgE or the membrane-anchored IgE on the surface of IgE-secreting plasma cells without risk of crosslinking IgE already bound on mast cells. The third approach is to block the action of the key cytokines, IL-4 or IL-5, involved in the chronic phase of inflammation or their receptors. Finally, the key roles of the adhesion molecules E-selectin and VLA-4 in eosinophil infiltration of tissues identifies these molecules as prime targets for antibody intervention.

4.9 Blood disorders

4.9.1 Hemolytic disease of the newborn

Hemolytic disease of the newborn is a life-threatening condition in which the erythrocytes of a fetus become lysed *in utero,* resulting in the birth of an infant with anemia and other disorders. The condition occurs when there is a maternal–fetal incompatibility in the expression of the red blood cell Rhesus D (RhD) antigen. If a mother is RhD –ve, and has previously become sensitized to the RhD antigen by an earlier RhD +ve pregnancy, she will produce antibody reactive with the RhD antigen when stimulated by RhD +ve fetal erythrocytes that pass through the placenta into her circulation. The maternal anti-RhD antibody is transported across the placenta, along with normal protective IgG, into the fetal circulation. Immunization can be prevented by the passive administration of anti-RhD antibody to the mother to block RhD antigen present on fetal cells that reach the maternal circulation at the birth of the first RhD +ve child (Section 5.7.1).

4.9.2 Idiopathic thrombocytopenic purpura

Idiopathic thrombocytopenic purpura (ITP) is a blood disorder characterized by abnormally low platelet counts. The disease manifests as episodes of bleeding, the severity of which correlates with the extent to which the number of platelets is decreased from normal levels. ITP is thought to be caused by the destruction of platelets by the immune system; autoantibodies that bind to platelet surface antigens, including gpIIb/IIIa (CD41/CD61) and gpIb/IX (CD42), destine them for destruction via Fc receptor-mediated phagocytosis by cells of the RES. The administration of large amounts of polyclonal Ig can significantly decrease platelet destruction by saturating the Fc receptor-dependent clearance mechanism and so alleviate the severity of ITP (Section 5.7.1).

4.10 Cardiovascular disease

The major types of cardiovascular disease – coronary artery thrombosis (heart attack), cerebrovascular thrombosis (stroke) and venous thrombosis – are caused by the blockage of critically sited blood vessels with consequent loss of blood flow to vital organs. The cause of blockage is thrombus, or clot, formation at the site of a ruptured atherosclerotic plaque in the blood vessel wall. Such thrombi are formed from cross-linked fibrin and frequently contain platelet-rich material.

In acute MI, blockage of the coronary artery damages the heart tissue and frequently leads to death. A method of treating acute infarction, and unstable angina symptomatic of atherosclerosis, is percutaneous transluminal coronary angioplasty (PTCA). In this procedure, a balloon catheter is introduced into the lumen of a clogged blood vessel and inflated at the site of blockage to open up the vessel by disintegrating the thrombus. A proportion of patients experience abrupt closure of the treated artery soon after angioplasty because of new thrombus formation and suffer subsequent ischemic damage (Section 4.8.2).

Blood vessels that become damaged by PTCA express tissue factor on the surface of their endothelial cells. Tissue factor triggers the coagulation cascade by converting factor VII to factor VIIa. The tissue factor–factor VIIa complex in turn activates factor X and factor Xa cleaves prothrombin. The thrombin generated by this sequence converts fibrinogen into fibrin which then polymerizes to form the clot. Mabs able to inhibit the action of tissue factor or the clotting factors VIIa and Xa, which act early in the cascade, may be able to inhibit the coagulation process and reduce the formation of new thrombi following angioplasty.

Platelets that adhere to sites of vascular injury are activated by thrombin which induces a conformational change in the integrin gpIIb/IIIa. The activated receptor can bind to a number of circulating adhesive molecules, principally fibrinogen. The result is the recruitment of further platelets through fibrinogen bridging and platelet aggregation. The activated gpIIb/IIIa molecule is a key target for antibody intervention because of its restriction to platelets and its principal role in the process of platelet aggregation during clot formation (Section 5.8). However, platelets play an important role in maintaining the integrity of blood vessels, and inhibition of their function diminishes their capacity to staunch bleeding from damaged vessels.

Another approach to treating MI is the use of thrombolytic agents, such as streptokinase, urokinase or tissue-type plasminogen activator, that activate fibrinolysis, dissolve occluding clots and restore blood flow. Antibody targeting of fibrinolytic agents to appropriate thrombus-specific antigens can improve their potency and selectivity. Target antigens that are absent from fibrinogen itself include the amino terminus of the β chain of fibrin and the fragment D-dimer, a cleavage product of cross-linked fibrin. Alternative targets in platelet-rich clots are cell-surface molecules such as gpIIb/IIIa and thrombospondin that distinguish the activated platelets in the clot from resting platelets in the circulation.

4.11 Neurological disorders

A number of neurological disorders, such as Alzheimer's disease, Parkinson's disease, Huntington's disease and amyotrophic lateral sclerosis, a type of motor neuron disease, are characterized by the degeneration of specific neuronal cells. The presence of tight junctions between the endothelial cells lining blood vessels in the brain, the blood–brain barrier (Section 1.6.3), limits the penetration of even small drugs from the systemic circulation to brain tissue and completely prevents the passage of polypeptides such as neurotrophic factors. Specific receptors exist on the luminal surface of the endothelium to transport certain ligands to the abluminal side by a process known as transcytosis. Iron, a necessary co-factor for enzymes that mediate various metabolic processes in the brain, is transported into the brain complexed with the protein carrier transferrin by transcytosis mediated via transferrin receptors. A Mab that binds to the transferrin receptor, which is abundantly present on endothelial cells throughout the brain, can transport nerve growth factor across the blood–brain barrier after injection into the peripheral circulation.

4.12 Wound healing

Wounds produced by surgery, trauma or burns often heal with the formation of disorganized scar tissue that results in the tightening of surrounding tissue and can lead to functional impairment or defective growth. Scarring is believed to reflect the overactivity of TGF-β which attracts inflammatory cells to the wound site and stimulates angiogenesis and the formation of extracellular matrix. Injection of a neutralizing Mab to TGF-β into the margins of healing dermal wounds can reduce the extent of inflammation and new blood vessel formation and restore a more normal skin architecture and tensile strength without inhibiting the rate of wound healing. A number of ophthalmic disorders, such as proliferative vitreoretinopathy, are characterized by excessive scar tissue formation in response to accidental or surgical trauma to the eye. Cellular hyperproliferation may be inhibited by targeting cytotoxic agents (Section 3.6) using Mabs that recognize a growth factor receptor, such as the transferrin receptor, that is preferentially expressed on the proliferating cells.

Chapter 5

Clinical studies of antibodies

5.1 Introduction

The success of antibody therapy depends upon the selection of target antigens which identify molecules or cells that are key participants in the pathogenesis of disease. Antibody that has been raised against the target antigen must be produced in quantity, purified to a high degree and extensively characterized in terms of molecular and antigen-recognition properties. The mode of action and potency of the antibody are investigated in cell or tissue assays *ex vivo* and in appropriate experimental animal models of disease. Pre-clinical studies aim to identify the factors that serve to limit antibody efficacy or give rise to unwanted side-effects and thereby help to define the most suitable strategies for antibody therapy. Importantly, pre-clinical studies form the scientific foundation for the testing of experimental antibody therapies in human clinical studies. Clinical trials seek to establish that a novel therapeutic antibody can be administered to patients safely and that the treatment has demonstrable and meaningful clinical benefit in the target disease indication. The ability to manufacture adequate amounts of antibody consistently and economically to the appropriate standard of quality underpins the ability to perform pre-clinical and clinical studies, to gain regulatory approval to market the product, and to satisfy the potential demand for a successful therapeutic.

5.2 Therapeutic antibody products

5.2.1 Polyclonal Ig

Polyclonal Ig is obtained from pools of human plasma (Section 2.2). The separation of Ig from other plasma constituents involves a process of selective precipitation. The fractionated antibody essentially consists of pure IgG, mainly monomer with smaller amounts of dimer and oligomer, trace amounts of other plasma proteins such as IgM and IgA, and antibody fragments. Immunoglobulin may be further purified by chromatographic procedures. The production of Ig from human donors carries with it the risk of transferring pathogens to the recipient. Accordingly, plasma donations that are used to make polyclonal Ig preparations are tested stringently to ensure that they are safe and free from known infectious viruses, in particular human immunodeficiency virus (HIV), hepatitis B virus (HBV) and hepatitis C virus (HCV). The traditional procedures for Ig fractionation are effective in eliminating HBV and HIV. Increasingly, Ig preparations are further subjected to solvent and detergent treatments that can eliminate HCV and other membrane-enveloped viruses without damaging the antibody. None the less, the possibility exists that novel infectious agents arising in the natural human population could break through the existing controls placed upon the purity of human Ig preparations.

5.2.2 Manufacture of Mabs

The process of Mab manufacture involves the fermentation of antibody-producing cells (Sections 2.3 and 2.4) followed by purification of the antibody product. Cell lines used for antibody manufacture are chosen for their ability to produce antibody of the appropriate target selectivity, antigen-binding avidity and isotype. In addition, to satisfy the criteria of bulk manufacture, the cell lines have to multiply sufficiently rapidly to seed large-scale culture, need to be stable expressors of antibody over the entire period of the manufacturing process, and must secrete the antibody at levels sufficient to provide the quantities required at economical cost. A master cell bank is created to contain multiple vials of frozen cells for long-term storage over the intended life-time of the antibody product. A manufacturer's working cell bank is derived from one of the master vials and individual lots used for each fermentation run.

Antibodies for initial clinical trials may be produced from hybridoma cells transplanted into mice or rats. Alternatively, antibody-producing cells can be maintained in high-density culture using hollow-fiber bio-reactors. Antibody-secreting cells are most commonly grown in low-density suspension culture within large stirred tanks or airlift fermenters. The supernatant from the fermentation broth is processed to purify the antibody product to the specified quality. The concentration of antibody, its physico-chemical characteristics, its ratio to the total protein in the supernatant and the nature of other components in the supernatant, all influence downstream processing. Generally, the supernatant is clarified by membrane filtration or centrifugation. The antibody may then be concentrated by ultrafiltration or ion-exchange chromatography. Finally, one or more steps of affinity chromatography may be included to achieve a higher level of purity. Immobilized protein A and protein G, which bind to the Fc regions of a variety of different isotypes, are especially useful for the purification of intact antibody.

5.2.3 Regulation of antibody products

Antibody-based therapeutics are controlled under the statutory regulations that apply to conventional pharmaceutical products to ensure quality, consistency, safety and efficacy. In the United States, antibody products are regulated by the Center for Biologics Evaluation and Research of the Food and Drug Administration. Approval to undertake trials requires submission of the details of pre-clinical research and a plan of proposed clinical studies in an Investigational New Drug application. The results of the clinical trials form part of a Product License Application that seeks approval to commence commercial sales of the product. The production of the antibody therapeutic is also regulated through an Establishment License Application and review of manufacturing facilities. Manufacture is carried out according to a Good Manufacturing Practice scheme that has been designed, implemented and controlled to guarantee the integrity of the antibody throughout the procedure, the quality of the final formulated product and the batch-to-batch reproducibility of the process.

The nature of an antibody-producing cell line, the manufacturing process, procedures for antibody purification and manipulation and the quality of the final product have to be stringently controlled and checked to satisfy regulatory authorities that a monoclonal or recombinant antibody is safe for testing in humans. The key objective of ensuring that the antibody is free from potentially harmful organisms or substances is met by testing for known or suspected contaminants and by developing and validating manufacturing and purification procedures that are designed to exclude or eliminate potential pathogens entirely. The final product has to be free from contamination by known bacteria, mycoplasma and fungi, viruses of murine, bovine or human origin, retroviruses and any type of adventitious virus. The levels of other contaminants, such as animal proteins, DNA, endotoxin and other pyrogens, constituents of culture media and components that may leach from chromatography columns, must be maintained within acceptable limits.

5.2.4 Pre-clinical studies

Pre-clinical studies are intended to provide detailed information about the antibody, demonstrate the scientific basis of its expected therapeutic activity and identify the likely incidence and severity of any potential side-effects.

The structural integrity of the antibody molecule is checked to demonstrate that it has not become fragmented, aggregated or otherwise modified. The avidity and specificity of binding of the antibody is preferably determined by direct binding to the purified target antigen. Appropriate positive and negative controls include at least one antibody of irrelevant antigen-binding specificity but similar isotype and a non-target antigen with similar physico-chemical properties to the actual target. The cross-reactivity of the antibody with normal human tissues is usually assessed by histochemical procedures using a battery of specified frozen tissues derived from a number of unrelated donors. Quantitative binding assays are used to ensure lot-to-lot consistency of antibody potency. Functional assays of potency in a biological model are important for quality control of antibodies, particularly if the assays can be correlated with mechanism of action and clinical efficacy. In the case of immunoconjugates (Section 2.6), there are additional requirements to satisfy relating to the other component(s) in the conjugate, the structure and purity of the product, and its immunoreactivity, potency and stability.

The efficacy of antibody therapy is established in pre-clinical studies by carefully controlled experiments in one or more animal species. Animal models seek to imitate the mechanistic, pharmacological or physiological characteristics of the disease in humans as closely as possible so as to demonstrate the principle of action, establish meaningful biological measures and identify optimal dosing schedules. Pre-clinical studies of antibodies can have limited value because experimental animals may not express a target antigen with the same epitope recognized by the experimental antibody, the antigen may be distributed differently on the tissues, or the antigen behaves differently to the human version. In addition, the experimental antibody may not interact with the animal's immune system in the way that it naturally engages human effector mechanisms. Nonhuman primates may be the most appropriate animal species in which to demonstrate efficacy in pre-clinical studies, although such studies are not generally considered to be mandatory.

Pharmacokinetic and biodistribution studies are essential to establish the serum half-life, rate of excretion and tissue localization of antibody in experimental animals. Pre-clinical studies in animals are important to understand the relationship between antibody behavior and efficacy *in vivo* and to compare the behavior of different antibody constructs. Short-term toxicology is commonly carried out in at least two different species, one of which may be a rodent, to measure hematological, biochemical or histopathological signs of toxicity and to identify sensitive organs and tissues. The unique properties of Ig molecules complicate the interpretation of traditional toxicity studies. Side-effects caused by interaction with human immune effector cells may not be adequately modeled in animals and the development of a humoral response to the experimental antibody can invalidate repeat dosing studies. Long-term studies of chronic toxicity, mutagenicity and teratogenicity may be conducted in parallel with clinical trials.

5.2.5 Clinical trials

Clinical trials are conducted in an ordered, lengthy and highly regulated process that passes through three distinct phases.

Phase I trials. Intended to make a preliminary evaluation of safety and pharmacology, phase I studies gradually escalate the dose of antibody to identify safely the maximal tolerated dose or the optimal biological dose and the dose-limiting toxicity. Trials are normally conducted in a limited number of healthy volunteers unless toxic side-effects are likely, when patients with the target disease are recruited. Additionally, phase I studies may provide preliminary evidence of biological activity, immunogenicity and therapeutic efficacy.

Phase II trials. The aim of phase II trials is to gather additional safety information and to provide preliminary evidence of efficacy. The studies generally explore the most appropriate dose, route and schedule of antibody administration and attempt to demonstrate the value of using particular measures, or end-points, of clinical utility. Reduced mortality is the most conclusive indicator of therapeutic efficacy in life-threatening diseases. Surrogate end-points that correlate with improvement in disease status, such as clinical or laboratory measurements, may be an accepted alternative where effects on survival would take too long to establish. Antibody treatment is preferably compared with a placebo, a harmless substance that is not expected to have any therapeutic effect. Whereas phase I trials are conducted as 'open-label' studies, phase II trials are preferably double-blinded and randomized to control for the occurrence of misleading results.

Phase III trials. The pivotal trials for drug approval are designed to demonstrate statistically significant evidence of clinical benefit in the targeted patient population measured using relevant end-points and controls. Antibody treatment is generally compared with placebo in diseases for which there is no satisfactory existing treatment or with active drug where there is already an approved treatment. In addition to establishing efficacy, phase III trials also accumulate further long-term safety data. In some instances, an approved product may be evaluated in further (phase IV) trials during which additional information on safety or efficacy considered desirable by the regulatory authorities is obtained.

Mixtures of antibody products can be regulated as a single product. 'Cocktails' contain two or more antibodies that are administered at a fixed ratio based on a clear rationale and the establishment of the efficacy of the components individually and in combination. 'Panels' consist of sets of antibodies directed against related antigens from which one or more members can be selected for use in each individual patient based on characterization of the patient's target antigen profile.

5.3 Immunodeficiency

Human polyclonal Ig has been administered for many years to patients with primary immunodeficiency (Section 4.5.1) to reduce the incidence of microbial infection by supplementing abnormally low levels of antibody. Ig preparations are known to contain antibodies that can block binding of microbes to target cells, opsonize microbes for phagocytosis and neutralize microbial toxins. Administration of polyclonal Ig by the intramuscular (im) route cannot produce serum levels of antibody within the normal range and has been superseded by intravenous (iv) Ig, or IVIG, as the standard form of therapy. The efficacy of several standard IVIG preparations has been supported by clinical studies in disease populations. IVIG preparations have also been approved for protection against opportunistic infection in secondary immunodeficiencies (Section 4.5.2) such as the bacterial infections that frequently occur in patients with B-cell chronic lymphocytic leukemia. Subcutaneous (sc) infusion can also achieve normal serum concentrations of Ig.

A number of side-effects are associated with the iv infusion of human Ig. Mild and reversible side-effects including headache, backache, flushing, chills, fever and nausea commonly occur soon after the first infusion, especially if the Ig is administered rapidly. In a small proportion of patients, an aseptic meningitis syndrome characterized by severe headache, fever, vomiting and signs of meningeal irritation may develop, resolving later when Ig administration has been discontinued. Anaphylactic reactions (Section 4.8.7) sometimes occur when Ig preparations, which contain small amounts of IgA, are infused into patients who are congenitally IgA-deficient.

5.4 Infectious disease

5.4.1 Viral diseases

Hyperimmune Ig preparations have been used for several decades in the prophylaxis of specific viral diseases caused by rabies virus, HBV and VZV (Section 4.6.1). The side-effects produced by hyperimmune Ig preparations appear similar to, and no more severe than, those associated with standard IVIG preparations. The efficacy of hyperimmune Ig in preventing serious CMV disease in immune-suppressed kidney transplant patients has been defined by randomized, double-blinded, placebo-controlled studies. IVIG preparations may also have efficacy in preventing CMV disease in patients who are undergoing liver trans-

Table 5.1: Antibody prophylaxis of respiratory syncytial virus disease

Agent	Hyperimmune human Ig
Antigen	Respiratory syncytial virus (RSV)
Disease	Premature infants, infants with bronchopulmonary dysplasia and infants with congenital heart disease at risk of RSV disease
Trial	Randomized phase III study (249 infants)
Protocol	150 mg kg^{-1} (low dose), 750 mg kg^{-1} (high dose), 3–5 iv infusions at 4-weekly intervals
Toxicity	Generally mild and rare, some cases of fluid overload, oxygen desaturation and fever
Efficacy	62% reduction in lower respiratory tract infection and 71% reduction in the severity of infection at the high dose

Reprinted by permission of *The New England Journal of Medicine*, Groothuis, J.R., Simoes, E.A.F., Levin, M.J. *et al.* (1993) Prophylactic administration of respiratory syncytial virus immune globulin to high-risk infants and young children. *New Engl. J. Med*, 330, 956–961.

plantation. Clinical trials have been conducted to measure the ability of monthly infusions of hyperimmune Ig to prevent or alleviate RSV infection in at-risk infants, based on animal studies and epidemiological evidence that correlated elevated anti-RSV levels with improved protection (*Table 5.1*). Infants that received a high dose of hyperimmune Ig had a reduced incidence and severity of RSV disease. In contrast, treatment of infants with established RSV infection was not found to be effective.

A number of human or humanized anti-viral Mabs are currently in development and entering phase I or phase II clinical trials. The use of high-affinity Mabs for prophylaxis may allow the delivery of neutralizing titers of antibody by the im route. However, Mabs react with only a single viral epitope and cocktails of Mabs may be necessary to ensure cross-reactivity with the majority of naturally occurring viral variants.

5.4.2 Bacterial sepsis

Experimental studies of anti-endotoxin antisera in various animal models of bacterial sepsis (Section 4.6.3) have demonstrated that the highest protective effect resides in the IgM fraction. However, extensive clinical trials of anti-lipid A IgM Mabs have so far failed to demonstrate unequivocal evidence of therapeutic efficacy in patients with sepsis. A mouse IgM Mab, E5, demonstrated some survival benefit in a subgroup of patients with sepsis who had not gone into refractory shock but this finding was not substantiated in a subsequent trial. Some patients showed an allergic response to E5 administration and a high proportion developed a human anti-mouse antibody (HAMA) response, although this did not seem to be associated with any untoward clinical consequences. In contrast, in trials of a human IgM Mab, HA-1A, there were no serious adverse reactions and no evidence of anti-HA-1A antibody responses. Phase III trials of HA-1A suggested an apparent benefit in patients with Gram-negative sepsis accompanied by shock, although this benefit could not be confirmed subsequently and mortality was apparently increased in sepsis patients without Gram-negative infection. Anti-TNF-α Mabs have also failed to show significant clinical benefit in sepsis patients in a number of clinical trials to date. The difficulties experienced in obtaining clear-cut proof of antibody efficacy in sepsis reflect the complex and diverse etiology and pathology of sepsis and suggest that assumptions about the biological roles of endotoxin and TNF-α based on the results of animal experiments may have been too simplistic.

5.5 Cancer

Animal models of cancer and metastasis have been used to investigate the feasibility of treating neoplasms with antibodies raised against numerous tumor-associated antigens (Section 4.7.1). Transplants of human tumors or tumor cell lines can grow without rejection as solid or disseminated tumors in mice and other rodents immune-suppressed by irradiation, in nude mice or in SCID mice. Treatments are generally most successful when antibody is administered before or simultaneously with tumor transplantation or when the established tumor burdens are small. Antigen-specific Mabs are more effective than polyclonal Ig preparations. Murine Mabs have been able to induce substantial and long-lasting tumor depletion in some mouse models, although more potent immunoconjugates are more reliably effective. In general, both Mabs and immunoconjugates have proved less effective against solid tumors than against leukemias and lymphomas.

5.5.1 Monoclonal antibodies

Pilot and phase I clinical trials of murine Mabs (Section 3.4.1) directed against a variety of target antigens have been undertaken in patients with hematological malignancies, including acute lymphocytic leukemia, chronic lymphocytic leukemia, B-cell lymphomas, T-cell leukemias and lymphomas, and myeloid neoplasms. The majority of patients treated in these studies had advanced disease refractory to prior chemotherapy and radiotherapy. Tumor responses were inconsistent and, in patients who responded to antibody therapy, most tumor regressions were either incomplete or of short duration. Target cells eliminated from the circulation became rapidly replaced by tumor cells from other organs including bone marrow or lymph nodes, once the Mab had cleared. Mabs unable to activate cell-mediated cytotoxicity generally failed to show clinically meaningful tumor responses. Toxicities resulting from iv in-

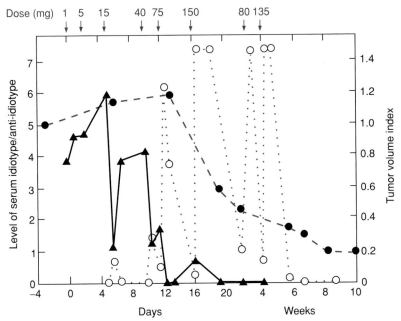

Figure 5.1: Effect of anti-idiotype Mab on level of serum idiotypic Ig and tumor volume; ▲, idiotype ($\mu g\ ml^{-1}$); ○ anti-idiotype ($\mu g\ ml^{-1} \times 10^{-1}$); ● tumor volume index. Reprinted by permission of *The New England Journal of Medicine*, Miller, R.A., Maloney, D.G., Warnke, R. and Levy, R. (1982) Treatment of B-cell lymphoma with monoclonal anti-idiotype antibody. *New Engl. J. Med.* **306**, 517–522.

fusion of mouse Mabs have usually been mild including fevers, chills, rashes, headaches, arthralgias, nausea and vomiting. More serious side-effects such as dyspnea, chest tightness, hypotension and cardiac arrhythmias occurred rarely. A number of complications, either singly or in combination, served to limit the efficacy of antibody therapy. The development of a HAMA response was a frequent occurrence that could inhibit retreatment with antibody. The properties of some target antigens limited the efficacy of therapy because antigenic modulation or shedding from the cell surface occurred (Section 4.7.1). Antigenic heterogeneity and limited access of antibody to solid tumor deposits also prevented more complete tumor eradication (Section 4.7.6).

Antibody therapy has shown occasional dramatic results in hematological malignancies. One patient with a B-cell-derived poorly differentiated lymphocytic lymphoma, which was progressing rapidly and failing to respond to drug and cytokine therapy, was treated with multiple infusions of a mouse Mab raised against the idiotype of the tumor surface Ig (Section 4.7.2). The patient entered into a complete remission that was durable for many years (*Figure 5.1*). Partial responses were also

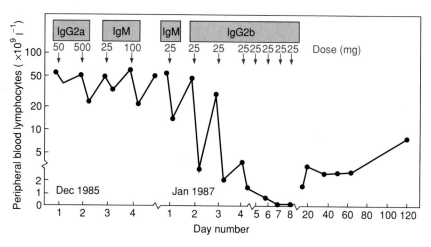

Figure 5.2: Effects of CAMPATH-1 rat Mabs of different isotype in a patient with B-cell chronic lymphocytic leukemia. Reproduced from Dyer, M.J.S., Hale, G., Hayhoe, F.G.J. and Waldman, H. (1989) Blood, **73**, 1431–1439, with permission from W.B. Saunders Company.

observed in a high proportion of other B-cell lymphoma patients treated with individually prepared anti-idiotypic mouse Mabs. Tumor regressions occurred relatively soon after Mab treatment, although solid tumor masses were observed to regress over a prolonged period, suggesting an active immune involvement. Side-effects were relatively innocuous and immune responses to the mouse Mab were rare because patients with advanced B-cell lymphoma are immune-suppressed by the disease. Trials in B-cell lymphoma highlighted a number of obstacles to antibody therapy. The majority of B lymphocyte tumors release significant amounts of surface Ig that can neutralize Mab before it reaches the tumor cells. A further problem was the emergence of tumor cell clones bearing mutant forms of the surface Ig that were able to evade the effects of treatment with a single anti-idiotypic Mab. The CD20 antigen, which is present on a high proportion of B-cell non-Hodgkin's lymphoma cells and is not subject to antigenic modulation or shedding, may be a superior target for antibody therapy. In preliminary dose-escalation studies, a human/mouse chimeric CD20 Mab, C2B8, induced tumor regressions after a single infusion.

The CD52 antigen is abundantly expressed on the surface of lymphoid cells, does not readily undergo modulation, and is a good target for complement-mediated cytotoxicity (Section 1.6.1). In patients with lymphoproliferative disorders, rat IgM and IgG2a versions of the CD52 Mab CAMPATH-1, which are able to activate complement but not to bind to human Fc receptor-bearing cells (Section 2.3.2), induced only transient falls in peripheral white blood cells. A rat IgG2b version, which was additionally able to bind to and activate human effector cells, depleted malignant cells from blood, marrow and spleen more efficiently (*Figure 5.2*). A humanized IgG1 version of the CAMPATH-1 Mab induced complete remission with recovery of normal hematopoiesis. CD52 Mab is less effective against tumor in lymph nodes and extra-nodal tumor masses, and ineffective when given intrathecally presumably because the cerebrospinal compartment lacks effector cells. Side-effects such as fevers, rigors and nausea were short-term. Host responses to the Mabs were absent probably because patients were immune suppressed by their disease and because the treatment itself depleted T lymphocytes. Adult T-cell leukemias constitutively express elevated levels of the high-affinity IL-2 receptor (Section 1.4.3). The mouse anti-Tac Mab, which does not activate human complement or ADCC, binds selectively to the α chain of the receptor and blocks the binding of IL-2. A significant number of patients treated with anti-Tac in a phase I trial developed tumor remissions although the majority subsequently relapsed and became unresponsive to further treatment. Following relapse, tumor cells continued to express the high affinity IL-2 receptor and to bind anti-Tac suggesting that they had progressed to an IL-2-independent growth status.

The most extensive clinical studies of a murine Mab targeted against a solid tumor have involved the mouse IgG2a Mab 17-1A that is capable of mediating ADCC with human effector cells (Section 1.6.2). 17-1A recognizes the epithelial membrane antigen (EMA) that is over-expressed by most tumor cells in the majority of colorectal cancer patients. Pilot clinical studies of 17-1A showed that the Mab was well tolerated. Occasional responses and remissions were observed in patients with advanced metastatic disease, although no consistent pattern of response or improvement in survival was evident. Interestingly, the onset of tumor regression was delayed until some time after antibody treatment had finished, implying an active immune response. A high proportion of patients receiving the mouse Mab developed an anti-idiotypic humoral response that mimicked the structure of the target antigen (Section 3.5). In colorectal carcinoma, metastatic tumor cells disseminated in mesenchymal and reticuloendothelial tissues are a good target for antibody therapy because they are relatively accessible to antibody in the bloodstream. A phase III trial of 17-1A in patients with minimal residual colorectal cancer (*Table 5.2*) showed a statistically significant reduction in mortality and a prolonged recurrence-free interval in patients receiving the antibody (*Figure 5.3*). The trial gave evidence for the prevention or the delay of the outgrowth of distant metastases though not of local recurrences. Side-effects were mild despite the fact that EMA is expressed by certain normal epithelial tissues (Section 5.5.4). Clinical trials of the 17-1A Mab using several different treatment protocols have identified a strong correlation between the

Table 5.2: Adjuvant antibody therapy of colorectal carcinoma

Agent	17-1A Mab (mouse IgG2a)
Antigen	Epithelial membrane antigen (EMA)
Disease	Colorectal carcinoma with spread to regional lymph nodes (Dukes' C classification) following surgical resection of tumor
Trial	Prospective, controlled, randomized phase III study (189 patients in total)
Protocol	500 mg, then four 100 mg doses at monthly intervals, iv infusion
Toxicity	Infrequent, mild constitutional symptoms, rare anaphylactic reactions
Immunogenicity	HAMA in 80% of patients after 2nd or 3rd infusion
Efficacy	30% reduction in mortality and 27% reduction in tumor recurrence in Mab-treated group at 5 years

Data compiled with permission from *The Lancet Ltd.* from Riethmuller, G., Schneider-Gadicke, E., Schlimot, G. *et al.* (1994) Randomized trial of monoclonal antibody for adjuvant therapy of respected Duke's C colorectal carcinoma. *Lancet, 343*, 1177–1183. © The Lancet Ltd., 1994.

occurrence of tumor regression and the activation of anti-anti-idiotype T cells capable of responding to cells bearing the EMA antigen.

Clinical studies of Mabs in patients with other solid tumors have been substantially less successful to date. Phase I clinical studies have demonstrated that mouse Mabs, which recognize the cell membrane gangliosides GD2 and GD3 and are able to activate complement and ADCC, can induce partial and complete responses in patients with advanced malignant melanoma and neuroblastoma. Mab administered by the iv

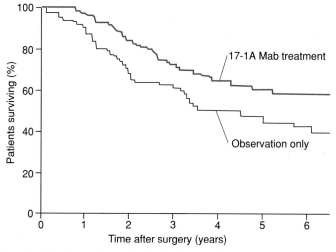

Figure 5.3: Overall survival of colorectal cancer patients treated with 17-1A Mab. Reprinted with permission from *The Lancet Ltd.*, Riethmuller, G., Schneider-Gadicke, E., Schlimok, G. *et al.* (1994) Randomised trial of monoclonal antibody for adjuvant therapy of respected Duke's C colorectal carcinoma. *Lancet, 343*, 1177–1183. © The Lancet Ltd., 1994.

route has been shown to localize at tumor sites, although different metastases within the same patient could regress, remain unchanged or progress in response to treatment. The responding tumor sites were characterized by evidence of complement deposition, lymphocyte infiltration and mast-cell activation. Side-effects were generally mild, with urticaria and pruritis prominent, and nausea, vomiting and diarrhea at the highest dose levels. However, treatment with a particular anti-GD2 Mab, 14G2a, of the mouse IgG2a isotype, was associated with significant toxic side-effects, including transient abdominal/pelvic pain, a delayed extremity pain syndrome and a reversible neuropathy.

5.5.2 Radioimmunoconjugates

Studies of radioimmunotherapy (RAIT) for the treatment of cancer have most commonly involved the use of radioimmunoconjugates incorporating β-particle emitters (Section 3.6.1). ^{131}I has a long history of use in the treatment of thyroid cancer and can be readily attached to antibody with retention of immunospecificity (Section 2.6.1). Of the metallic radionuclides, ^{90}Y has been the best investigated to date. In animal tumor models, the selective localization of radioimmunoconjugate in tumor sites can be demonstrated and therapeutic effects are evidenced by tumor shrinkage or outright cure. In contrast with animal studies, trials of radioimmunoconjugates in cancer patients have been much less successful to date because toxic side-effects have limited the doses that could be administered.

The dose-limiting toxicity of systemic RAIT is to the bone marrow and severe myelosuppression occurs at doses of radiation that are generally suboptimal for tumor eradication. A number of approaches can be adopted to limit the risk of damage to the bone marrow. An unlabeled antibody can be administered to complex with and accelerate the clearance of the excess radiolabeled antibody from the bloodstream via less radiosensitive organs. Low-dose external irradiation or hyperthermia applied to the tumor site can increase capillary permeability specifically in the region of the tumor so that more of the administered dose reaches its target. Another option, locoregional delivery, involves the injection of radioimmunoconjugate directly into body cavities within which the tumor is known to be localized (Section 3.9.1). Compared with systemic injection, locoregional delivery diminishes toxicity to the bone marrow and other radiosensitive organs or tissues and can directly expose the tumor to higher doses of radiation. Alternatively, the myeloablative effects of high-dose RAIT can be mitigated by the concurrent administration of bone marrow-sparing cytokines or bone marrow transplantation (Section 4.3).

Tumor regressions have been reported with both ^{131}I- and ^{90}Y-labeled antibodies in a number of preliminary clinical studies, although the responses have generally proved to be only partial and transient. The best clinical results with RAIT have been observed in studies of leukemias and lymphomas that are highly radiosensitive and are present in the vascular compartment where they are readily accessible to radio-immunoconjugate administered by the iv route. Objective tumor regressions have been documented in patients with chronic lymphocytic leukemia, cutaneous T-cell lymphoma, non-Hodgkin's lymphoma and Hodgkin's disease. Conventional chemotherapy can cure approximately half of the patients with high- or intermediate-grade B-cell lymphomas but few, if any, with low-grade B-cell lymphoma. High-dose chemotherapy in conjunction with bmt can cure up to half of the patients who have relapsed, but the remainder relapse for a second time. Impressive evidence of efficacy has been observed in phase I trials of patients receiving radioimmunoconjugates targeted to the CD20 antigen at doses of conjugate that are not myeloablative (*Table 5.3*). Trace-labeled antibody was used to estimate the dose of unlabeled Mab giving the highest ratio of tumor localization relative to normal tissue. Interestingly, tumor responses were observed during the tracer studies, indicating that the naked antibody was itself inducing anti-tumor effects (Section 5.5.1). A higher rate still of long-lasting remissions has been seen in patients receiving larger doses of radioimmunoconjugate combined with bone marrow rescue (*Table 5.4*). In general, patients with smaller tumor burdens appeared more likely to show favorable antibody biodistribution and experience tumor responses.

In trials of systemic RAIT in patients with more radioresistant tumors, such as melanoma, neuroblastoma and colorectal carcinoma, only sporadic regressions have generally been seen in patients with advanced and refractory disease. A high proportion of partial remissions and some complete remissions were observed in hepatoma patients who were treated iv with ^{131}I- and ^{90}Y-labeled polyclonal antibodies or Mabs directed against ferritin in combination with conventional radiotherapy

Table 5.3: Radioimmunotherapy of B-cell lymphoma

Agent	[^{131}I]Anti-B1 Mab (mouse IgG2a)
Antigen	CD20 antigen
Disease	B-cell lymphoma refractory to chemotherapy
Trial	Phase I dose-escalation study
Protocol	Administration of tracer doses and gamma camera imaging 15 mg therapeutic dose (34–66 mCi) iv
Toxicity	Mild or no myelosuppression
Immunogenicity	HAMA in 2/9 patients
Efficacy	6/9 tumor responses including 4/9 complete remissions lasting 8 to >11 months

Reprinted by permission of *The New England Journal of Medicine*, Kominski, M.S., Zasadny, K.P., Francis, I.R. *et al.* (1993) Radioimmunotherapy of B-cell lymphoma with [131I] anti-B1 (anti-CD20) antibody. *New Engl. J. Med.* **329**,459–465.

Table 5.4: Radioimmunotherapy of B-cell lymphoma with autologous bone marrow support

Agents	^{131}I-labeled mouse IgG2a Mabs B1, IF5 or mouse IgG1 Mab MB-1
Antigen	CD20 antigen (B1, IF5) or CD37 antigen (MB-1)
Disease	B-cell lymphoma refractory to chemotherapy
Trial	Phase I dose-escalation study
Protocol	Administration of tracer doses and gamma camera imaging 58–1168 mg therapeutic dose (234–777 mCi) iv Autologous bone marrow reinfusion
Toxicity	Myelosuppression, nausea, minor infections, some cases of cardiopulmonary toxicity
Efficacy	19/19 tumor responses, including 2/19 partial remissions and 16/19 complete remissions, 9 in continuous remission for 3–53 months

Reprinted by permission of *The New England Journal of Medicine*, Press, O.W., Eary, J.F., Appelbaum, F.R. (1993) *et al.* Radiolabeled-antibody therapy of B-cell lymphoma with autologous bone marrow support. *New Engl. J. Med.* **329**,1219–1224.

or chemotherapy. Locoregional RAIT has been explored in the treatment of several solid tumor types. ^{131}I-labeled Mabs recognizing neuroblastoma and carcinoma TAAs have been administered intrathecally to patients with neoplastic meningitis and objective responses seen. Complete and partial remissions were observed in patients with glioblastoma who were treated by intratumoral administration of ^{131}I-labeled Mab. In ovarian carcinoma patients, neoplastic disease is often restricted to the peritoneal cavity. The targeting of free-floating malignant cells is greatly enhanced by administration of antibody by the intraperitoneal (ip) route. Although patients with large ip tumor nodules show poor responses, patients with microscopic disease can apparently be rendered disease-free for extended periods of time using ^{90}Y-labeled immunoconjugates made with the HMFG1 Mab recognizing the polymorphic epithelial mucin (PEM), an antigen expressed by many epithelial cancers (*Table 5.5*). In these clinical studies, human antibody responses were regularly observed against both the mouse Mab and a series of different metal-ion chelators. Evidence for the activation of both humoral and cellular responses suggested that triggering of anti-idiotypic networks (Section 1.4.6) may have contributed to the observed clinical effects.

5.5.3 Immunotoxins

Clinical trials of systemic immunotoxin therapy were first conducted with antibody–ricin A chain conjugates (Section 3.6.3). In patients with melanoma, breast carcinoma and colorectal carcinomas, disease stabilization or transient mixed responses were observed in a proportion of patients following a single course of therapy and there was one complete response. The tumor regressions observed occurred over a matter

Table 5.5: Adjuvant radioimmunotherapy of ovarian carcinoma

Agent	^{90}Y-HMFG1 Mab (mouse IgG1)
Antigen	Polymorphic epithelial mucin (PEM)
Disease	Ovarian carcinoma following surgery and chemotherapy
Trial	Pilot phase I/II studies
Protocol	25 mg dose (5–30 mCi) ip
Toxicity	Reversible myelosuppression depending on chelating agent
Immunogenicity	HAMA (100%), anti-chelator responses
Efficacy	19/21 patients surviving with no evidence of residual disease at 3–62 months (median 35 months)

Reprinted by permission of Wiley-Liss, Inc., a subsidiary of John Wiley & Sons, Inc. from Hird, V., Maraveyas, A., Snook, D. *et al*. Adjuvant therapy of ovarian cancer with radioactive monoclonal antibody. *Br. J. Cancer*, **68**, 403–406.

of months following immunotoxin therapy, suggesting that host immune responses had been triggered. Toxic symptoms, which were generally tolerable and fully reversible, included malaise, loss of appetite, mild fevers, chills, myalgia and arthralgia, and mild hepatic and neurological abnormalities. The dose-limiting toxicity was a capillary or vascular leak syndrome characterized by a fall in total serum protein, fluid shifts, weight gain and peripheral edema. The most severe toxicity reported was a severe and prolonged neuropathy that occurred in patients who received an immunotoxin that cross-reacted with Schwann cells and caused nerve cell demyelination. In the majority of patients, an antibody response against both the murine Mab and the toxin A chain developed.

Trials with more promising results have been conducted in lymphoma patients using immunotoxins targeted to B-cell differentiation antigens (Section 1.4.2). Tumor responses were observed in patients receiving a ricin A chain immunotoxin targeted against the CD22 antigen (*Table 5.6*). The presence of a large antigen load on tumor cells readily accessible in the circulation resulted in the rapid adsorption of immunotoxin and protected against the development of the capillary leak syndrome.

Table 5.6: Immunotoxin therapy of B-cell lymphoma

Agent	Mouse IgG1 Mab RFB4–deglycosylated ricin A chain immunotoxin
Antigen	CD22 antigen
Disease	B-cell lymphoma resistant to conventional therapy
Trial	Phase I dose-escalation study
Protocol	2–12 iv infusions at 2 day intervals (4.7–142 mg m^{-2} total)
Toxicity	Vascular leak syndrome, myalgia
Immunogenicity	9/24 anti-immunotoxin responses
Efficacy	1/24 complete and 5/24 partial remissions lasting 30–78 days

Data compiled from Amlot, P.L., Stone, M.J., Cunningham, D. *et al*. (1993) A phase I study of an anti-CD22-deglycosylated ricin A chain immunotoxin in the treatment of B-cell lymphoma resistant to conventional therapy. *Blood*, **82**, 2624–2633, with permission from W.B. Saunders Company.

Table 5.7: Adjuvant immunotoxin therapy of B-cell lymphoma

Agent	Mouse IgG1 Mab anti-B4–blocked ricin immunotoxin
Antigen	CD19 antigen
Disease	B-cell lymphoma in complete remission following autologous bmt
Trial	Phase I dose-escalation study
Protocol	20–50 μg kg^{-1} day^{-1} for 7 days, continuous iv infusion
Toxicity	Transient elevation of hepatic enzymes and reversible thrombocytopenia, mild capillary leak syndrome
Immunogenicity	7/12 anti-immunotoxin responses
Efficacy	11/12 complete remissions lasting 13–26 months (median 17 months) post-transplantation

Data compiled from Grossbard, M.L., Gribben, J.G., Freedman, A.S. *et al.* (1993) *Blood*, **81**, 2263–2271, with permission from W.B. Saunders Company.

A similar pattern of toxic effects and responses was observed with an analogous A chain immunotoxin prepared with the Fab′ fragment of the same Mab. A blocked ricin immunotoxin recognizing the CD19 antigen has been used in the treatment of refractory B-cell lymphoma. Significant anti-tumor responses, including complete remissions, were observed especially in patients with low tumor burdens. Relapse in non-Hodgkin's lymphoma is primarily attributable to clones of lymphoma that are resistant to high-dose therapy. Autologous bmt permits drug or radiation treatment regimens to be intensified and can overcome tumor cell resistance, but the procedures for purging bone marrow often fail to remove all contaminating tumor cells. An alternative is to target residual tumor cells with immunotoxin *in vivo* after bmt. In this situation of minimal residual disease, a high proportion of lymphoma patients experienced durable remissions with blocked ricin immunotoxin therapy (*Table 5.7*). In studies of both types of immunotoxin, the toxic side-effects were reversible and a proportion of patients developed an antibody response to both the toxin and antibody components of the immunotoxin.

5.5.4 Chemoimmunoconjugates

Clinical studies with antibody–drug conjugates (Section 3.6.2) have been undertaken in patients with lung and colon carcinoma and neuroblastoma. Side-effects were generally found to be mild, including rash, chills and fever. In general, there was little or no evidence of significant tumor responses. In one case, patients treated systemically with a vinca alkaloid immunoconjugate in a phase I/II study developed an acute inflammatory lesion of the duodenal mucosa leading to epigastric pain, nausea, vomiting and diarrhea. The immunoconjugate, made with the mouse IgG2a Mab KS1/4, recognizing EMA, cross-reacted with normal human tissue and activated complement so leading to inflammation. The side-effect was not observed in studies using chimpanzees, although biopsy studies did show localization of the chemoimmunoconjugate to the duodenum. The antibody component acted as a hapten carrier system and, in addition to HAMA, a humoral response against the conjugated drug occurred.

5.5.5 Anti-idiotypic Mabs

The potential of anti-idiotypic Mabs (Section 3.5) in cancer has been investigated in a few clinical trials. Preliminary studies of a mouse IgG1 Mab MK2-23, which mimics the melanoma HMW-MAA, have demonstrated the general safety of subcutaneous (sc) delivery, with side-effects being limited to flu-like symptoms, arthralgias and myalgias even upon repeated administration. The mouse Mab stimulated a HAMA response and an anti-idiotypic response in patients. One complete remission and some minor responses were observed in a preliminary clinical trial. A human IgG1 anti-idiotypic Mab 105AD7, which mimics the gp72 antigen associated with colorectal tumor, has been administered sc to patients in a phase I trial. There was no evidence of toxicity and anti-tumor antibodies were not detected. However, a cellular response to immunization with the Mab was indicated by the detection of IL-2 in plasma and the capacity of patients' T lymphocytes to proliferate on exposure to gp72 antigen-positive cells. The anti-idiotype Mab extended the median time of survival of colorectal cancer patients compared with a contemporary group of patients who did not receive Mab treatment (*Figure 5.4*).

5.5.6 Bispecific antibodies

The first clinical trials of effector cell retargeting (Section 3.4.2) used bispecific antibody constructs with specificity for the CD3 antigen in combination with autologous T lymphocytes activated with cytokines *ex vivo* for locoregional tumor therapy. Ovarian carcinoma patients who received an ip infusion of activated T cells armed with a bispecific antibody recognizing a tumor-surface antigen experienced local tumor regressions and mild toxicity. In contrast, a preliminary study of systemic treatment found that the administration of a bispecific antibody targeting the CD3 antigen was associated with severe toxicity, involving fevers, chills, headache, fatigue and hypotension thought to be mediated via TNF-α released by activated T cells in the circulation.

Phase I studies have been conducted with a quadroma-derived mouse IgG1 bispecific Mab (Section 2.3.3), with dual specificity for FcγRIII and the HER-2 antigen that is over expressed by a significant proportion of breast and ovarian carcinomas. The bispecific Mab demonstrated immune activation when administered iv to patients with breast carcinoma. Minor and mixed clinical anti-tumor responses were observed. The treatment was associated with significant release of TNF-α, IL-6 and IL-8, leading to fever and rigors, and a dose-limiting thrombo-

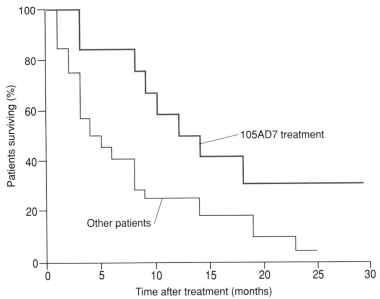

Figure 5.4: Survival of colorectal cancer patients treated with anti-idiotypic Mab 105AD7. Reprinted by permission of Wiley-Liss, Inc., a subsidiary of John Wiley & Sons, Inc., Deuton, G.W.L., Durrant, L.G., Hardcastle, J.D., Austin, E.B., Sewell, H.F. and Robins, R.A., (1994) Clinical outcome of colorectal cancer patients treated with human monoclonal anti-idiotypic antibody. *Int. J. Cancer*, **57**, 10–14.

cytopenia in some patients. Initial clinical trials have been conducted with another bispecific antibody made by chemical coupling (Section 2.6.2) of an anti-HER-2 mouse Fab′ fragment and a mouse Fab′ fragment able to bind to FcγRI at a site outside the Fc-binding site that is usually occupied by endogenous IgG. Rapid binding to, and activation of, monocytes was observed shortly after iv infusion of the bispecific Fab′ dimer. Tumor regressions were observed, including a partial remission with eradication of multiple metastases. Immune activation increased the plasma levels of TNF-α, IL-6 and G-CSF, although cytokine release was associated with only mild fevers and chills.

5.6 Transplantation

Preparations of polyclonal Ig raised in rabbits or horses, such as anti-thymocyte globulin (ATG), are powerful immunosuppressive agents that have a history of use in treating allograft rejection (Section 4.8.5). Polyclonal Ig preparations tend to give rise to serum sickness (Section 1.7.2) and side-effects that are caused by the nonspecific binding of antibody to nonlymphocytic blood cells and to other normal human tissues. A number of Mabs directed against T-cell-specific surface antigens have

Table 5.8: Monoclonal antibody reversal of acute kidney transplant rejection

Agent	OKT3 Mab (mouse IgG2a)
Antigen	CD3 antigen
Disease	Acute rejection of cadaveric renal transplants
Trial	Prospective, randomized phase III study of Mab (combined with a reduction in the dosage of concomitant immunosuppressive medication) versus conventional high-dose steroid treatment (123 patients in total)
Protocol	5 mg iv dose daily for 1–28 days (14 days mean)
Toxicity	Cytokine release syndrome
Immunogenicity	HAMA in 80% of patients during or after the 2nd week of treatment
Efficacy	OKT3 reversed 94% of rejections compared with 75% for steroids
	One-year graft survival of 62% in OKT3-treated group versus 45% in the control group

Reprinted by permission of *The New England Journal of Medicine*, Ortho Multicenter Transplant Study Group (1985) A randomized clinical trial of OKT3 monoclonal antibody for acute rejection of cadaveric renal transplants. *New Engl. J. Med.*, **313**, 337–342.

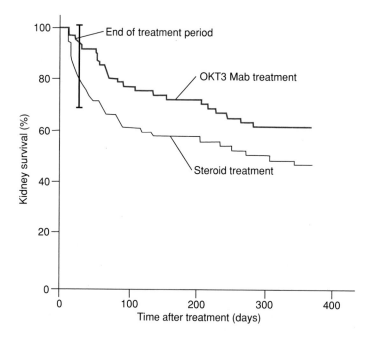

Figure 5.5: Kidney survival in patients receiving OKT3 Mab treatment for acute renal allograft rejection. Reprinted by permission of *The New England Journal of Medicine*, Ortho Multicenter Transplant Study Group (1985) A randomized clinical trial of OKT3 monoclonal antibody for acute rejection of cadaveric renal transplants. *New Engl. J. Med.*, **313**, 337–342.

been developed to act as immunosuppressive agents by blocking T-cell function.

5.6.1 OKT3 Mab

OKT3 is a mouse Mab directed against the CD3 antigen that is present on all mature T lymphocytes of humans and higher primates (Section 1.4.3). OKT3 induces a profound immune suppression during administration but not long-term tolerance. Rapid clearance of CD3 +ve T cells from the circulation occurs within the first few hours following iv administration of the Mab. A proportion of T cells are opsonized and removed by Fc-binding cells of the RES. Other T cells bind the Mab and antigenic modulation removes the CD3 antigen from the cell surface. CD3 +ve cells remain undetectable provided that the level of circulating OKT3 is maintained by continued administration. When administration is discontinued, CD3 +ve cells reappear rapidly and reach normal levels within 1 week.

In a pivotal phase III clinical trial, OKT3 was shown to be more effective at reversing the acute rejection of donor kidney transplants in patients than conventional high-dose steroid treatment when used as first-line therapy (*Table 5.8*). Patients treated with OKT3 in first rejection responded to Mab treatment within 20 days of the start of treatment, whereas the responses were delayed in the case of rescue treatments involving steroid- or ATG-resistant rejection episodes. Kidney survival 1 year after the onset of treatment was higher in the case of OKT3 (*Figure 5.5*), although there was no significant difference in the rates of subsequent rejection episodes. Further clinical trials have demonstrated the ability of OKT3 to reverse acute rejection of hepatic, cardiac and combined kidney–pancreas transplants. The value of OKT3 has also been demonstrated in prophylactic, or induction, therapy when the Mab is administered in conjunction with other immunosuppressive agents immediately following transplantation to prevent or substantially delay the occurrence of first acute rejection episodes.

Administration of OKT3 is frequently associated with a spectrum of systemic flu-like side-effects. The so-called 'cytokine release syndrome' includes fevers, chills, dyspnea, chest pain and tightness, wheezing, diarrhea, nausea and vomiting. The side-effects are common upon the first administration of OKT3 and are easily controlled in most patients. The process of Mab binding transiently activates T cells and causes them to release relatively large amounts of cytokines, such as TNF-α, IFN-γ, IL-2, IL-3 and IL-6, which are believed to mediate the side-effects of this first-dose syndrome. The side-effects no longer occur once CD3 +ve T cells have been completely eliminated following two or three infusions. More severe side-effects, such as aseptic meningitis and pulmonary edema, can occur in some patients and necessitate intensive care. The T-cell-activating properties of OKT3 result from cross-linking of the CD3-associated TCR via Fcγ receptor-bearing cells that interact with the Fc region of cell-bound OKT3. Mutant recombinant CD3 Mabs that cannot bind to Fc receptors with high affinity no longer activate T cells yet retain their immunosuppressive properties (Section 2.7.1).

The prolonged administration or repeated use of OKT3, especially in combination with other immune suppressants, can lead to excessive immune suppression and put patients at risk of contracting serious viral diseases or lymphoproliferative disorders. Most patients receiving OKT3 develop a HAMA response, although this generally does not prevent subsequent readministration of the Mab. Anti-idiotypic responses that can neutralize antibody are also frequent and high titers may preclude useful administration of a second dose of OKT3. The incidence of human antibody responses can be reduced by concurrent administration of other immunosuppressive agents, by shortening the time period over which OKT3 is administered, or by substituting OKT3 with a humanized CD3 Mab.

5.6.2 Anti-T-cell Mabs

T-cell activity can be blocked by Mabs that recognize key functional surface antigens other than CD3 (Section 1.4.3). Rodent Mabs directed against the TCR demonstrate similar efficacy to OKT3 in reversing allograft rejection when used as primary therapy. However, anti-TCR Mabs appear not to deplete peripheral T cells as extensively as the CD3 Mab OKT3. BMA031 is a mouse IgG2b Mab directed against a common epitope of the α/β TCR. In a phase III blinded, randomized clinical trial of induction immunosuppression in renal transplantation, the anti-TCR Mab significantly reduced the incidence of rejection events that occurred within the first 10 days after transplantation. There were no serious side-effects of the treatment. Although the anti-TCR Mab induced the release of TNF-α, the release of this cytokine alone failed to trigger the first-dose syndrome characteristic of OKT3 (Section 5.6.1). A HAMA response to BMA031 developed extremely rapidly. Preliminary clinical studies of a rat IgG2a Mab, 33B3.1, recognizing the α subunit of the IL-2 receptor, demonstrated that the Mab was as effective as ATG in preventing acute rejection after first transplantation but was not successful in reversing ongoing rejection episodes. The Mab was well tolerated, although a high proportion of patients developed both anti-isotypic and anti-idiotypic responses. Humanized Mabs directed against either the α or β chain of the IL-2 receptor (anti-Tac and Mik β1 respectively) have been shown to prolong the survival of cardiac allografts in primates and to be less immunogenic than their murine counterparts.

5.7 Immune-mediated disorders

5.7.1 Intravenous Ig

Numerous clinical studies have indicated that IVIG may be of therapeutic benefit, at least in a proportion of patients, in a variety of different inflammatory and autoimmune diseases (Section 4.8). However, there have been relatively few controlled clinical trials. The mechanisms of action of polyclonal Ig in these disorders are not fully understood and appear to be complex. Ig preparations contain antibodies that can block the action of cytokines, inhibit T-cell activation and proliferation and suppress autoantibody production by anti-idiotypic interaction. In addition some of the effects observed may have been mediated by non-Ig components.

IVIG has been shown to be of value in the treatment of blood disorders (Section 4.9). In patients with idiopathic thrombocytopenic purpura (ITP), treatment with IVIG induces either partial or complete responses as evidenced by transient or persistent normalization of platelet counts. Several lines of evidence indicate that IVIG exerts a major part of its effects by blocking Fc receptors present on the cells of the RES that are responsible for the elimination of platelets coated with autoantibody. Hyperimmune Ig against the Rhesus D (RhD) antigen is predominantly used to prevent immunization of RhD −ve pregnant women by red blood cells of a RhD +ve fetus. Anti-RhD antibody preparations have also been used to treat ITP patients who are RhD +ve, under the rationale that red blood cells coated with anti-RhD antibody can compete for capture by RES cells and saturate the uptake mechanism, thereby sparing platelets. A potential side-effect of anti-RhD antibodies is excessive destruction of erythrocytes, with risk of anemia.

5.7.2 Anti-TNF Mab

TNF-α is a major regulatory cytokine involved in the pathogenesis of arthritis (Section 4.8.4). In animal models of collagen-induced arthritis, anti-TNF Mabs achieved a significant reduction in disease pathology even when administered after the development of severe arthritis. A mouse/human chimeric Mab, cA2, which combines mouse V domains and a human IgG1 framework, and so is able to both fix complement and bind to cellular Fc receptors, has been studied in clinical trials. In a phase I/II open-label trial of cA2 in patients with long-standing disease, significant decreases in the levels of blood markers of inflammation, such as C-reactive protein, were detected. Improvements were seen in clinical assessments of disease activity, such as morning stiffness, pain and number of swollen joints. In a subsequent double-blinded, placebo-controlled trial in patients with active rheumatoid arthritis refractory to other treatments, there was a significant dose-dependent improvement

Table 5.9: Monoclonal antibody treatment of rheumatoid arthritis

Agent	cA2 mouse/human IgG1 chimeric Mab
Antigen	TNF-α
Disease	Active rheumatoid arthritis refractory to conventional treatment
Trial	Double-blind, randomized, placebo-controlled phase II study (73 patients in total)
Protocol	1 mg kg^{-1} or 10 mg kg^{-1} iv infusion
Toxicity	Minor side-effects, some infections
Efficacy	Paulus 20% response at week 4 in 19/24 at high dose and 11/25 at low dose compared with 2/24 for placebo
	Paulus 50% response at week 4 in 14/24 at high dose compared with 2/24 for placebo

Data compiled with permission from *The Lancet Ltd.*, Elliot, M.J., Maini, R.N., Feldmann, M.*et al.* (1994a) Repeated therapy with immoclonal antibody to tumor necrosis factor *alpha* (cA2) in patients with rheumatoid arthritis. *Lancet*, **344**, 1125–1127. © The Lancet Ltd., 1994.

in clinical status according to measures of the Paulus index, an amalgam of six clinical, observational and laboratory variables (*Table 5.9*). Treatment with cA2 was well tolerated: the most common side-effect appeared to be an increase in the incidence of minor infections, although this was not clearly related to the dose of Mab. In responding patients, the effect of Mab treatment lasted several months before relapse occurred. In patients who experienced a disease flare, repeat treatment with cA2 resulted in further good clinical responses (*Figure 5.6*). Human antibody responses specific for the murine sequences of cA2 developed in half of the patients who underwent retreatment but did not block the biological action of the Mab.

5.7.3 Anti-T-cell Mabs

Several open-label, nonrandomized clinical trials have been undertaken in patients with rheumatoid and psoriatic arthritis, using mouse and mouse/human chimeric Mabs recognizing the CD4 antigen (Section 1.4.3). In some patients, improvements in clinical symptoms occurred within the first month after treatment and lasted for several weeks or months. Treatment with the chimeric Mab M-T412 induced a rapid and prolonged depression in the number of circulating CD4 +ve T cells. Favorable clinical responses were related not to lymphocyte counts but to the circulating level of unbound Mab, suggesting that the observed therapeutic effects may have been determined by the extent to which Mab was able to penetrate into the synovial sites of inflammation. Side-effects were generally minor and correlated with an elevation in the serum level of IL-6 but not TNF-α. Anti-idiotypic responses were frequently observed.

A phase I clinical trial has also been undertaken in patients with refractory rheumatoid arthritis using CAMPATH-1H, the humanized

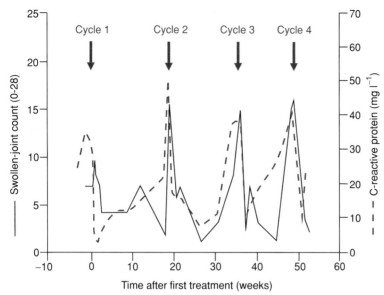

Figure 5.6: Responses to four successive cycles of cA2 Mab in a patient with rheumatoid arthritis. Reprinted with permission from *The Lancet Ltd.*, Elliot, M.I., Maini, R.N., Feldman, M. *et al.* (1994b) Randomised double-blind comparison of chimeric monoclonal antibody to tumour necrosis factor *alpha* (cA2) versus placebo in rheumatoid arthritis. *Lancet*, **344**, 1105–1110. © The Lancet Ltd., 1994.

version of the CD52 Mab with a human IgG1 isotype (Section 5.5.1). The first infusion of Mab induced a rapid decrease in lymphocyte counts that remained suppressed for several months after treatment. Clinical improvements were observed and the responses sustained for several months. Transient fever, rigors and nausea developed in all patients upon administration of the first dose of CAMPATH-1H. After a single course of therapy, there was no measurable anti-Mab response. However, three of four patients who were retreated with the humanized Mab, including those who shared the identical allotype, developed an antibody response against the idiotype of the Mab. Preliminary studies have sought to explore the effects of combination treatment with humanized CD52 and CD4 Mabs in autoimmune disease.

A variety of antibodies directed against T cells, including ATG, murine anti-T-cell Mabs and a ricin A chain immunotoxin against the CD5 antigen, have been investigated for the treatment of acute graft-versus-host disease (GVHD) (Section 4.8.6). A feature of these trials has been a high incidence of relapse in treated patients and an increased risk of infectious complications resulting from the immunodeficiency induced by T-cell depletion. A pilot clinical study of a mouse IgG1 Mab, BT563, directed against the α chain of the IL-2 receptor, was undertaken in children with inherited diseases of the marrow receiving partially matched, T-cell-depleted bone marrow transplants. Patients that developed steroid-resistant acute GVHD received early and prolonged treatment with the Mab. A high proportion exhibited complete or partial responses. About half of the responders relapsed but could be put in second remission by a further course of Mab treatment. In a phase I/II study of a humanized version of the anti-Tac Mab (Section 5.5.1), approximately 40% of a mixed population of patients with steroid-resistant acute GVHD following allogeneic bmt responded to one or two treatments with Mab. Most responders later developed chronic GVHD and four died of pneumonia.

5.8 Acute ischemia

The Fab fragment of a mouse/human chimeric Mab, c7E3, binds to the gpIIb/IIIa receptor on platelets, blocks its function, and prevents the platelet aggregation that leads to blood clotting (Section 4.10). The Fab fragment has been administered to patients to prevent abrupt closure of an artery that can occur following angioplasty procedures (*Table 5.10*). A phase III prospective, randomized, double-blind trial demonstrated a significant reduction in the incidence of ischemic complications following angioplasty. Pre-clinical and pilot clinical studies had indicated that, to generate sufficient anti-thrombotic effects, it was necessary to block practically all the gpIIb/IIIa receptors present on circulating platelets, thereby impairing their hemostatic function. In the phase III trial, the incidence of bleeding episodes was increased at the sites of vascular

Table 5.10: Monoclonal antibody fragment prevention of acute ischemia

Agent	c7E3 mouse/human chimeric Fab fragment
Antigen	gpIIb/IIIa (CD41/CD61 antigens)
Disease	Prevention of acute ischemia following PTCA
Trial	Prospective, randomized, double-blind, placebo-controlled phase III study (2099 patients in total) – EPIC (Evaluation of 7E3 for the Prevention of Ischemic Complications) Study
Protocol	1. 0.25 mg kg^{-1} bolus 10 min before PTCA, infusion of 0.6 mg h^{-1} for up to 12 h 2. 0.25 mg kg^{-1} bolus, then placebo infusion 3. placebo bolus, placebo infusion
Toxicity	Increased rate of major bleeding complications and blood transfusion especially in bolus + infusion of Fab fragment
Efficacy	35% reduction in ischemic complications (death, MI, repeat PTCA) at 30 days post-angioplasty and 23% reduction in number of major ischemic events after 6 months in the bolus + infusion Fab-treated group compared with placebo

Data compiled with permission of The *New England Journal of Medicine* from The EPIC Investigators (1994) Use of a monoclonal antibody directed against the platelet glycoprotein IIb/IIIa receptor in high-risk coronary angioplasty. *New Engl. J. Med.*, **330**, 956–961.

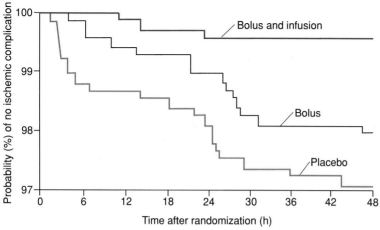

Figure 5.7: Effects of c7E3 Fab fragment on inhibiting the onset of nonfatal ischemic events requiring repeat angioplasty. Reprinted by permission of *The New England Journal of Medicine*, The EPIC Investigators (1994) Use of a monoclonal antibody directed against the platelet glycoprotein IIb/IIIa receptor in high-risk angioplasty. *New Engl. J. Med.*, **330**, 956–961.

puncture and coronary artery bypass grafting, but there was no evidence for an increase in the more serious complication of intracranial bleeding. Bolus injection followed by infusion produced the best protective effects, indicating the importance of inhibiting platelet function rapidly and for a sustained period of time (*Figure 5.7*). Humoral responses against the chimeric Fab fragment occurred less frequently in this trial than in pilot studies of a murine 7E3 Fab fragment which showed a positive serum anti-mouse Ig activity in about half of the patients treated.

5.9 The state of the art

The exploration of multiple experimental approaches in the clinic has helped to define both the advantages and limitations of different strategies in antibody therapy. In common with other types of pharmaceutical drug or therapeutic procedure, the theoretical and experimental arguments in favor of a particular antibody therapeutic have not always translated into a practical and effective treatment, especially when the target disease concerned has been complex, well-established or extensive. For any disease, several antigens represent possible targets that can be addressed using different antibodies with unique properties, a number of different therapeutic strategies and a variety of clinical protocols. In consequence, it is difficult to compare the results of clinical trials employing different antibody agents directly. Nevertheless, it is possible to draw a number of broad conclusions relevant to the current state of the art.

Target diseases. Antibody therapy has a clear role to play in preventing disease by supplementing natural immunity. Antibody treatments appear to be most valuable and to show most promise in acute and life-threatening situations when other options are not available or largely inadequate, other therapies have failed leaving progressive disease unchecked, or when therapeutic procedures put the patient's life at risk. In cases where partially or temporarily effective treatments exist, antibody therapy is most clearly useful as an adjunct to treatment, in situations of minimal residual disease, or in early relapse, rather than as single-agent first-line therapy.

Target antigens. Antigens that are principally or substantially involved in the mechanisms of pathogenesis, or that identify normal or abnormal cell types involved in the disease process, have been identified in a number of important diseases. The majority of the target antigens have complex molecular structures against which it has been possible to raise selectively binding antibodies. The favored targets for successful antibody therapy are extracellular or cell surface antigens that are directly accessible in the bloodstream or can be readily reached from the site of antibody administration.

Therapeutic strategies. The choice of therapeutic strategy is dictated by the biological characteristics of the target disease. Polyclonal Ig preparations, hyperimmune Ig, murine Mabs, chimeric Mabs and antibody Fab fragments have all demonstrated important therapeutic effects when used at doses that substantially or completely saturate target antigen sites. In cancer, conventional Mabs able to activate the effector arm of the immune system have generally failed to demonstrate significant anti-tumor activity, necessitating the continued exploration of more complex, more powerful and better-directed single- and two-stage antibody targeting strategies. Despite the apparent inadequacy of immune activation, there is tantalizing evidence that important immune-regulatory mechanisms may be triggered by both antibodies and immunoconjugates.

Toxic side-effects. Antibody drugs are generally well tolerated with mild, short-term and reversible side-effects. Certain side-effects are apparently unavoidable because they occur as the direct consequence of the intended biological action of the treatment. In some cases, more serious side-effects occur in patients whose medical complications are exacerbated by a treatment that is otherwise well tolerated. In other cases, unpredictable toxicities can occur as a result of the unintended cross-reaction of the antibody agent with normal tissues. As with other forms of therapy, the balance of therapeutic benefits against harmful side-effects has to be established independently for each agent in controlled clinical trials.

Immune side-effects. Anaphylactic reactions to antibody administration have been rare and are mostly avoidable. In the majority of patients, other than those who are severely immune-suppressed, a human antibody response occurs to any nonhuman parts of an antibody molecule and to the non-Ig components of immunoconjugate molecules. The clinical implications of such responses appear to be minor and the action of the antibody therapeutic is often left unaffected. The factors that determine the propensity to develop an anti-idiotypic response, which can block the action of readministered antibody, are not well understood. Whereas some murine Mabs elicit only weak responses, even humanized Mabs can stimulate a significant anti-idiotypic response.

5.10 The future

The time to convert a discovery or new technology into an approved and marketable product is typically 10–15 years. A gap of 10 years separated the invention of the hybridoma approach to the generation of Mabs in 1975 and the first definitive demonstration of the therapeutic efficacy of a mouse Mab (OKT3) in the clinic. A further decade elapsed before the approval of a chimeric antibody fragment (c7E3). The next 10 or 15 years promise the emergence of further important and novel antibody drugs. Future advances in antibody therapy are likely to stem from developments in antibody technology and from an improved understanding of the behavior of antibody molecules in humans.

Genetic engineering. The manipulation of Ig genes is proving to be an invaluable tool in refining antibody therapy. Humanized Mabs appear to be less immunogenic than their rodent counterparts and may allow for more prolonged or repeated treatment. Recombinant antibody fragments and fusion proteins offer enormous flexibility to tailor precisely the properties of antibody molecules and thereby to optimize their therapeutic activity. The development of antibodies with novel antigen binding specificities is likely to be accelerated by phage antibody technology.

Targeting and delivery. Antibody drugs are large protein molecules, the properties of which restrict their delivery to parenteral routes of administration, inhibit their ready access to certain tissues and organs in the body and block their ability to enter cells. The limitations to access and action may be mitigated by using recombinant antibodies with novel properties, two-stage targeting approaches that minimize side-effects and maximize therapeutic effects, and genetic approaches to antibody gene expression within cells.

Immune regulation. Fundamental research is describing in increasing detail the molecular and cellular mechanisms by which the immune system keeps disease at bay or contributes to it. An improved understanding of immune mechanisms may allow immune-activating Mabs, antibody conjugates or fusion proteins to be used for the immune regulation of disease. Given the apparent safety of many therapeutic antibodies, it may prove feasible to use antibody treatment in patients before their disease has developed to an advanced stage or they are subjected to other potentially harmful therapies.

In conclusion, antibody technology represents a rational, and readily applicable, approach to the development of novel therapeutic agents. Antibody drugs with unique biological actions can be generated. Clinical trials with antibody therapeutics have demonstrated that they can be both safe and efficacious in certain types of medical application. Moreover, antibody trials have helped to confirm the role of a number of target antigens and cell types in human disease and identified them as viable biological targets for therapy.

Appendix A. Glossary

Abzyme: an antibody molecule like an enzyme that is capable of catalyzing a chemical reaction (also *Catalytic antibody*).

Adjuvant: a substance that enhances the immune response to an immunogen.

Affinity maturation: the increase in the affinity of antigen-specific antibodies during an antibody response.

Allergen: an antigen that stimulates a hypersensitive or allergic immune reaction.

Alloantigen: a foreign or non-self antigen.

Allotype: the antigenic characteristics of antibodies determined by allelic polymorphisms that differ between individuals of the same species.

Allotypic determinant: an antigenic determinant distinguishing different allotypes.

Anaphylaxis: an acute and potentially life-threatening allergic reaction to a systemically administered foreign protein, characterized by disseminated inflammation.

Anergy: a state of cellular unresponsiveness to antigenic stimulation (see also *Tolerance*).

Antibody: a type of soluble globular protein produced by the B lymphocytes of the immune system in response to antigenic stimulation (also *Immunoglobulin*).

Antibody affinity: the strength of binding between an antigen and a single antigen-combining site of an antibody molecule (see also *Antibody avidity*).

Antibody avidity: the overall strength of binding between a bivalent or polyvalent antibody molecule and a multimeric antigen or an antigen array (see also *Antibody affinity*).

Antibody cocktail: a therapeutic antibody preparation comprising a mixture of two or more antibodies in a fixed ratio (see also *Antibody panel*).

Antibody conjugate: an antibody molecule to which another antibody molecule or a nonantibody component has been attached by chemical procedures (also *Immunoconjugate*, see also *Antibody fusion protein*).

Antibody fragment: a portion of an antibody generated by proteolysis or genetic engineering that is structurally intact and retains its physiological function.

Antibody fusion protein: a recombinant antibody molecule the structure of which is specified by fusing gene segments that encode one or more antibody domains and a nonimmunoglobulin polypeptide (see also *Antibody conjugate*).

Antibody mimetic: an oligopeptide or nonpeptide molecule that mimics the antigen-binding characteristics of an antibody by resembling the structure of complementarity-determining regions.

Antibody molecule: an antibody, antibody analog, antibody derivative or antibody fragment.

Antibody panel: a collection of antibodies directed against related antigens from which one or more members can be selected for individualized patient therapy (see also *Antibody cocktail*).

Antibody response: the induction of antigen-specific antibody production in response to stimulation of the immune system by an immunogen (also *Humoral immune response*).

Antigen: a molecule that interacts with an antibody molecule via the antigen-combining site of the variable region.

Antigen-combining site: the portion of the variable region of an antibody molecule that binds the antigen.

Antigen presentation: the process by which protein antigens are converted into peptides and displayed in association with major histocompatibility complex molecules on the surface of antigen-presenting cells to activate T lymphocytes.

Antigenic determinant: the structural region of an antigen that is recognized by an antibody molecule (also *Epitope*).

Antigenic heterogeneity: the expression of different levels of an antigen by individual cells in a population of target cells.

Antigenic modulation: the disappearance of cell surface antigens that have been cross-linked by antibody via an active internalization process.

Antigenized antibody: a recombinant antibody in which one or more complementarity-determining regions have been substituted with peptide epitopes derived from a target antigen.

Anti-idiotypic antibody: an antibody that binds to the idiotypic region of another antibody molecule.

Anti-idiotypic response: the antibody response to the unique idiotypic determinants of antibody when administered to humans (see also *HAMA response*).

Antiserum: the fluid fraction of the blood that contains immunoglobulins.

Autoantibody: an antibody that binds to an autoantigen.

Autoantigen: an antigen in the body to which the immune system is normally tolerant (also *Self antigen*).

Bispecific antibody: an antibody with two antigen-combining sites each capable of recognizing a different antigen.

Bivalent antibody: an antibody molecule with two identical antigen-combining sites (see also *Univalent antibody*).

Carrier: an immunogenic protein that can stimulate an immune response against a nonimmunogenic antigen to which it is attached (see also *Hapten*).

Catalytic antibody: see *Abzyme*.

Chain shuffling: a method for creating novel antigen-combining sites by combinatorial pairing of variable domains from libraries of heavy- and light-variable genes using phage display.

Chemoimmunoconjugate: an immunoconjugate made by the chemical attachment of a chemotherapeutic drug to an antibody molecule.

Chimeric monoclonal antibody: a recombinant antibody that comprises variable domains derived from one animal species and constant domains derived from another species, usually human.

Class/Subclass: immunoglobulin type determined by the structure of the heavy chains (also *Isotype*).

Class switching: the expression of antigen-specific immunoglobulin with altered isotype by a clone of activated B lymphocytes.

Combinatorial library: a collection of variable domain gene pairings between multiple heavy chain and multiple light chain genes in random combination.

Complementarity-determining regions: the regions of polypeptide structure in the antigen-combining site that make physical contact with the antigen.

Constant gene/domain/region: constant gene exons encode individual constant domains that combine to form the constant regions of immunoglobulin molecules (see also *Variable gene/domain/region*).

Cytokine: a soluble protein molecule involved in signaling between cells.

Diabody: a heterodimeric recombinant antibody molecule with two antigen-combining sites formed by paired variable domains on different chains.

Dimeric antibody: an engineered antibody molecule comprising two immuno-globulin monomers covalently linked by chemical conjugation or genetic manipulation.

Epitope: see *Antigenic determinant.*

Epitope imprinted selection: a procedure that uses antigenic selection of phage antibodies and chain shuffling to direct the replacement of the original variable domains of an antibody while retaining its antigen-binding characteristics.

Fab arm: the antigen-binding portion of an IgG antibody that consists of a light chain and the amino-terminal portion of a heavy chain linked by a disulfide bond (see also *Fc region*).

Fc receptor: a cell-surface receptor recognizing the Fc region of an antibody.

Fc region: the portion of an IgG antibody that consists of the carboxy-terminal halves of the two heavy chains linked by the disulfide bonds of the hinge region and is responsible for interactions with other components of the immune system (see also *Fab arm*).

Framework regions: the regions of an antibody variable domain that are of relatively invariant amino acid sequence and form the scaffold for the hypervariable regions (see also *Hypervariable regions*).

HAMA response: the antibody response to mouse antibody when administered to humans directed against the common murine determinants (see also *Anti-idiotypic response*).

Hapten: an antigen that is not immunogenic unless attached to a protein carrier (see also *Carrier*).

Heterohybridoma: a hybridoma cell line made by fusing a heteromyeloma cell line and a human antibody-expressing B lymphocyte (also *Trioma*).

Heteromyeloma: a myeloma cell line made by fusing a human lymphoid tumor line and a mouse myeloma cell line.

Hinge region: a flexible nonglobular portion of the antibody heavy chains that allows movement of the Fab arms and Fc region relative to one another.

Humanization: the genetic replacement of the constant domains and framework regions of an animal antibody by human equivalents corresponding to grafting the complementarity-determining regions of an animal antibody on to a human framework.

Humanized monoclonal antibody: a recombinant version of a monoclonal antibody originally derived from an immunized animal that has undergone a humanization procedure (see also *Human monoclonal antibody*).

Human monoclonal antibody: a monoclonal antibody derived from an immortalized human antibody-expressing B-lymphocyte (see also *Humanized monoclonal antibody*).

Humoral immune response: see *Antibody response.*

Hybrid hybridoma: a hybrid cell line made by fusing two different hybridoma cell lines and capable of expressing a bispecific monoclonal antibody (also *Quadroma*).

Hybridoma: a hybrid cell line made by fusing a myeloma cell line and an antibody-expressing B lymphocyte and capable of continuous production of monoclonal antibody.

Hyperchimerization: a method of antibody humanization that employs computer modeling to predict changes in framework regions designed to optimize the conformation of the grafted complementarity-determining regions.

Hyperimmune immunoglobulin: the polyclonal antibody isolated from antiserum that contains elevated levels of antigen-specific immunoglobulin following vaccination.

Hypervariable regions: the regions of an antibody variable domain that display considerable variation in amino acid sequence and form the complementarity-determining regions (see also *Framework regions*).

Idiotope: an antibody epitope determined by a unique structural feature of the variable region (also *Idiotypic determinant*).

Idiotype: the antigenic characteristics of antibodies determined by differences in idiotopes.

Idiotypic determinant: see *Idiotope.*

Immune complex: the noncovalent complex formed by the interaction of one or more antibody and antigen molecules.

Immunization: the deliberate stimulation of an active immune response by exposure to an immunogen (see also *Vaccination*).

Immunoadhesin: an antibody fusion protein in which the antigen-binding variable regions have been replaced with a nonantibody ligand-binding protein molecule (see also *Immunoligand*).

Immunoconjugate: see *Antibody conjugate.*

Immunogen: an antigen that can stimulate an active immune response in an animal.

Immunoglobulin: see *Antibody.*

Immunoligand: an antibody fusion protein in which the antigen-binding variable regions have been replaced with a nonantibody polypeptide ligand (see also *Immunoadhesin*).

Immunoliposome: a liposome endowed with antigen-binding specificity by antibody attached to its surface.

Immunolysin: an antibody molecule combined with a membrane-acting protein toxin.

Immunotherapy: the treatment of disease by active stimulation of the immune system or by passive administration of components of the immune system such as antibodies and cytokines, or immune cells.

Immunotoxin: an antibody molecule combined with a naturally-occurring toxin or engineered toxin analog.

Immunovirus: a virus expressing antigen-binding variable domains of antibody on its surface.

Inflammation: the body's natural protective response to infection or injury, involving the activation of leukocytes and their infiltration into affected tissues.

Intravenous immunoglobulin: a preparation of polyclonal antibody formulated for intravenous administration.

Isotype: see *Class/Subclass.*

Miniantibody: a bivalent antibody molecule comprising univalent recombinant antigen-binding fragments dimerized via amphipathic helix interaction.

Minibody: a novel antigen-binding protein mimicking a portion of an antibody variable domain.

Monoclonal antibody: a unique antibody derived from a single clone of antibody-expressing B lymphocytes following immortalization or hybridoma formation (see also *Polyclonal antibody*).

Murine monoclonal antibody: a monoclonal antibody derived from an antibody-expressing B lymphocyte of a mouse or rat.

Myeloma: a tumor of plasma cells.

Neoantigen: a new antigenic determinant created by the linkage of two molecules.

Opsonization: the promotion of phagocytosis mediated by the binding of antibodies and complement fragments to the surface of a target cell.

Phage antibody: an antibody molecule with antigen-binding capacity expressed on the surface of a bacteriophage.

Phage display: the use of recombinant bacteriophage to express functional non-phage polypeptides on the surface of the virion.

Plasma cell: the antibody-secreting cell that represents the final stage of B cell maturation.

Polyclonal antibody: a mixture of antibodies derived from multiple clones of antibody-secreting plasma cells and isolated from serum (see also *Monoclonal antibody*).

Primatized monoclonal antibody: a chimeric antibody comprising variable domains derived from a nonhuman primate species and human constant domains.

Quadroma: see *Hybrid hybridoma.*

Radioimmunoconjugate: an antibody molecule to which a radionuclide has been attached by chemical procedures.

Recombinant monoclonal antibody: a monoclonal antibody derived from a cell line expressing recombinant immunoglobulin genes.

Reshaping: a method of antibody humanization that substitutes framework residues iteratively to optimize the conformation of the grafted complementarity-determining regions.

Resurfacing: a method of antibody humanization that maintains the conformation of the complementarity-determining regions by substituting the surface amino acid residues of the framework regions.

Self antigen: see *Autoantigen.*

Single domain antibody: an isolated heavy or light chain variable domain with antigen-binding properties.

Superantigen: a microbial protein that activates T cells by cross-linking major histocompatibility complex class II and T cell receptor molecules independently of antigen.

Surface immunoglobulin: the membrane-bound immunoglobulin that is expressed on the surface of B lymphocytes.

Tolerance: the programed failure of the immune response to respond to certain antigens, in particular, autoantigens.

Transfectoma: a myeloma cell line into which recombinant immunoglobulin genes have been transfected to express a recombinant antibody molecule.

Trioma: see *Heterohybridoma.*

Univalent antibody: an antibody molecule with a single functional antigen-combining site (see also *Bivalent antibody*).

Vaccination: the deliberate stimulation of an active immune response to a disease-related antigen for therapeutic purposes (see also *Immunization*).

Variable gene/domain/region: variable gene exons encode individual variable domains that combine to form the variable regions of immunoglobulin molecules (see also *Constant gene/domain/region*).

Xenogeneic antibody: an antibody derived from a foreign animal species.

Appendix B. Further reading

Reference books

Baldwin, R.W., Byers, V.S. and Mann, R.D. (eds.) (1990) *Monoclonal antibodies and immunoconjugates.* The Parthenon Publishing Group, Carnforth.

Borrebaeck, C.A.K. (1991) *Antibody engineering.* Oxford University Press, Oxford.

Borrebaeck, C.A.K. and Larrick, J.W. (eds.) (1990) *Therapeutic monoclonal antibodies.* Stockton Press, New York.

Epenetos, A.A. (ed.) (1991) *Monoclonal antibodies: applications in clinical oncology.* Chapman & Hall Medical, London.

Epenetos, A.A. (ed.) (1992) *Monoclonal antibodies 2: applications in clinical oncology.* Chapman & Hall Medical, London.

Fanger, M.W. R.G. (1995) *Bispecific antibodies.* Landes Company, Austin, TX.

Frankel, A.E. (ed.). (1988) *Immunotoxins.* Kluwer Academic Publishers, Dordrecht.

Goldenberg, D.M. (1994) *Cancer therapy with radiolabeled antibodies.* CRC Press, Boca Raton, FL.

Jencks, W.P. (1991) *Catalytic antibodies.* John Wiley Ltd., Chichester.

Liddell, J.E. and Weeks, I. (1995) *Antibody technology.* BIOS Scientific Publishers Ltd., Oxford.

Mayforth, R.D. (1993) *Designing antibodies.* Academic Press, New York.

Perkins, A.C. and Pimm, M.V. (1991) *Immunoscintigraphy: practical aspects and clinical applications.* Wiley-Liss, New York.

Rodwell, J.D. (ed.) (1988) *Antibody-mediated delivery systems.* Marcel Dekker, Inc., New York.

Sedlacek, H.-H., Seemann, G., Hoffmann, D., Czech, J., Lorenz, P., Kolar, C. and Bosslet, K. (1992) *Antibodies as carriers of cytotoxicity.* Karger, Basel.

Sedlacek, H.-H., Schulz, G., Steinstraesser, A., Kuhlmann, L., Schwarz, A., Seidel, L., Seemann, G., Kraemer, H.-P. and Bosslet, K. (1988) *Monoclonal antibodies in tumor therapy.* Karger, Basel.

Vogel, C.-W. (ed.) (1987) *Immunoconjugates: antibody conjugates in radio-imaging and therapy of cancer.* Oxford University Press, Oxford.

Waldmann, H. (ed.) (1988) *Monoclonal antibody therapy.* Karger, Basel.

Zola, H. (ed.) (1995) *Monoclonal antibodies: the second generation.* BIOS Scientific Publishers Ltd., Oxford.

Reference papers

Alegre, M.-L., Peterson, L.J., Xu, D. *et al.* (1994) A non-activating "humanized" anti-CD3 monoclonal antibody retains immunosuppressive properties *in vivo. Transplantation*, **57**, 1537–1543.

Amlot, P.L., Stone, M.J., Cunningham, D. *et al.* (1993) A phase I study of an anti-CD22-deglycosylated ricin A chain immunotoxin in the treatment of B-cell lymphomas resistant to conventional therapy. *Blood*, **82**, 2624–2633.

Anasetti, C., Hansen, J.A., Waldmann, T.A. *et al.* (1994) Treatment of acute graft-versus-host disease with humanized anti-Tac, an antibody that binds to the interleukin-2 receptor. *Blood*, **84**, 1320–1327.

Arteaga, C.L., Winnier, A.R., Poirier, M.C. *et al.* (1994) $p185^{c-erbB-2}$ signaling enhances cisplatin-induced cytotoxicity in human breast carcinoma cells: association between an oncogenic receptor tyrosine kinase and drug-induced DNA repair. *Cancer Res.*, **54**, 3758–3765.

Bagshawe, K.D., Sharma, S.K., Springer, C.J. and Antoniw, P. (1995) Antibody directed enzyme prodrug therapy: a pilot-scale clinical trial. *Tumor Targeting*, **1**, 17–29.

Barbas, C.F. III, Bain, J.D., Hoekstra, D.M. and Lerner, R.A. (1992) Semi-synthetic combinatorial antibody libraries: a chemical solution to the diversity problem. *Proc. Natl Acad. Sci., USA*, **89**, 4457–4461.

Batra, J.K., Kasturi, S., Gallo, M.G. *et al.* (1993) Insertion of constant region domains of human IgG1 into CD4–PE40 increases its plasma half-life. *Mol. Immunol.*, **30**, 379–386.

Baud, F.J., Sabouraud, A., Vicaut, E. *et al.* (1995) Treatment of severe colchicine overdose with colchicine-specific Fab fragments. *N. Engl. J. Med.*, **332**, 642–645.

Berthiaume, F., Reiken, S.R., Toner, M., Tompkins, R.G. and Yarmush, M. L. (1994) Antibody-targeted photolysis of bacteria *in vivo. Biotechnology*, **12**, 703–706.

Biocca, S., Pierandrei-Amaldi, P., Campioni, N. and Cattaneo, A. (1994) Intracellular immunization with cytosolic recombinant antibodies. *Biotechnology*, **12**, 396–399.

Bolt, S., Routledge, E., Lloyd, I. *et al.* (1993) The generation of a humanized, non-mitogenic CD3 monoclonal antibody which retains *in vitro* immunosuppressive properties. *Eur. J. Immunol.*, **23**, 403–411.

Bosslet, K., Czech, J. and Hoffmann, D. (1994) Tumor-selective prodrug activation by fusion protein-mediated catalysis. *Cancer Res.*, **54**, 2151–2159.

Brooks, P.C., Montgomery, A.M.P, Rosenfeld, M. *et al.* (1994) Integrin $\alpha_v\beta_3$ antagonists promote tumor regression by inducing apoptosis of angiogenic blood vessels. *Cell*, **79**, 1157–1164.

Cantarovich, D., Le Mauff, B., Hourmant, M. *et al.* (1994) Prevention of acute rejection episodes with an anti-interleukin 2 receptor monoclonal antibody. *Transplantation*, **57**, 198–203.

Caron, P.C., Jurcic, J.G., Scott, A.M., *et al.* (1994) A phase Ib trial of humanized monoclonal antibody M195 (anti-CD33) in myeloid leukemia: specific targeting without immunogenicity. *Blood*, **83**, 1760–1768.

Crowe, J.E. Jr., Murphy, B.R., Chanock, R.M., Williamson, R.A., Barbas, C.F. III and Burton, D.R. (1994) Recombinant human respiratory syncytial virus (RSV) monoclonal antibody Fab is effective therapeutically when introduced directly into the lungs of RSV-infected mice. *Proc. Natl Acad. Sci. USA*, **91**, 1386–1390.

Davies, J. and Riechmann, L. (1995) Antibody VH domains as small recognition units. *Biotechnology*, **13**, 475–479.

Debré, M., Bonnet, M.-C., Fridman, W.-H. *et al.* (1993) Infusion of Fcγ fragments for treatment of children with acute immune thrombocytopenic purpura. *Lancet*, **342**, 945–949.

Denton, G.W.L., Durrant, L.G., Hardcastle, J.D., Austin, E.B., Sewell, H.F. and Robins, R.A. (1994) Clinical outcome of colorectal cancer patients treated with human monoclonal anti-idiotypic antibody. *Int. J. Cancer*, **57**, 10–14.

Dohlsten, M., Abrahmsen, L., Björk, P. *et al.* (1994) Monoclonal antibody-superantigen fusion proteins: tumor-specific agents for T-cell-based tumor therapy. *Proc. Natl Acad. Sci. USA*, **91**, 8945–8949.

Duenas, M. and Borrebaeck, C.A.K. (1994) Clonal selection and amplification of phage displayed antibodies by linking antigen recognition and phage replication. *Biotechnology*, **12**, 999–1002.

Durrant, L.G., Buckley, T.J.D., Denton, G.W.L., Hardcastle, J.D., Sewell, H.F. and Robins, R.A. (1994) Enhanced cell-mediated tumor killing in patients immunized with human monoclonal antiidiotypic antibody 105AD7. *Cancer Res.*, **54**, 4837–4840.

Dyer, M.J.S., Hale, G., Hayhoe, F.G.J. and Waldmann, H. (1989) Effects of CAMPATH-1 antibodies *in vivo* in patients with lymphoid malignancies: influence of antibody isotype. *Blood*, **73**, 1431–1439.

Elliott, M.J, Maini, R.N., Feldmann M. *et al.* (1994a) Repeated therapy with monoclonal antibody to tumour necrosis factor α (cA2) in patients with rheumatoid arthritis. *Lancet*, **344**, 1125–1127.

Elliott, M.J., Maini, R.N., Feldman, M. *et al.* (1994b) Randomised double-blind comparison of chimeric monoclonal antibody to tumour necrosis factor *alpha* (cA2) versus placebo in rheumatoid arthritis. *Lancet*, **344**, 1105–1110.

The EPIC Investigators (1994) Use of a monoclonal antibody directed against the platelet glycoprotein IIb/IIIa receptor in high-risk coronary angioplasty. *N. Engl. J. Med.*, **330**, 956–961.

Evans, T.J., Moyes, D., Carpenter, A., *et al.* (1994) Protective effect of 55- but not 75-kD soluble tumor necrosis factor receptor-immunoglobulin G fusion proteins in an animal model of Gram-negative sepsis. *J. Exp. Med.*, **180**, 2173–2179.

Fagerberg, J., Hjeln, A.-L., Ragnhammar, P., Frodin, J.-E., Wigzell, H. and Mellstedt, H. (1995) Tumor regression in monoclonal antibody-treated patients correlates with the presence of anti-idiotype-reactive T lymphocytes. *Cancer Res.*, **55**, 1824–1827.

Farges, O., Ericzon, B-G., Bresson-Hadni, S., *et al.* (1994) A randomized trial of OKT3-based versus cyclosporine-based immunoprophylaxis after liver transplantation. *Transplantation*, **58**, 891–898.

French, R.R., Hamblin, T.J., Bell, A.J., Tutt, A.L. and Glennie, M.J. (1995) Treatment of B-cell lymphomas with combination of bispecific antibodies and saporin. *Lancet*, **346**, 223–224.

Gram, H., Marconi, L.-A., Barbas, C.F.III, Collet, T.A., Lerner, R.A. and Kang, A.S. (1992) *In vitro* selection and affinity maturation of antibodies from a naïve combinatorial immunoglobulin library. *Proc. Natl Acad. Sci. USA*, **89**, 3576–3580.

Green, L.L., Hardy, M.C., Maynard-Currie, C.E. *et al.* (1994) Antigen-specific human monoclonal antibodies from mice engineered with human Ig heavy and light chain YACs. *Nat. Genet.*, **7**, 13–21.

Greenman, R.L., Schein, R.M.H., Martin, M.A. *et al.* (1991) A controlled clinical trial of E5 murine monoclonal IgM antibody to endotoxin in the treatment of Gram-negative sepsis. *J. Amer. Med. Assoc.*, **266**, 1097–1102.

Griffiths, A.D., Malmqvist, M., Marks, J.D., *et al.* (1993) Human anti-self antibodies with high specificity from phage display libraries. *EMBO J.*, **12** 725–734.

Groothuis, J.R., Simoes, E.A.F., Levin, M.J. *et al.* (1993) Prophylactic administration of respiratory syncytial virus immune globulin to high-risk infants and young children. *N. Engl. J. Med.*, **329**, 1524–1530.

Grossbard, M.L., Gribben, J.G., Freedman, A.S. *et al.* (1993) Adjuvant immunotoxin therapy with anti-B4–blocked ricin after autologous bone marrow transplantation for patients with B-cell non-Hodgkin's lymphoma. *Blood*, **81**, 2263–2271.

Haug, C.E., Colvin, R.B., Delmonico, F.L. *et al.* (1993) A phase I trial of immunosuppression with anti-ICAM-1 (CD54) mAb in renal allograft recipients. *Transplantation*, **55**, 766–773.

Hawkins, R.E., Russell, S.J. and Winter, G. (1992) Selection of phage antibodies by binding affinity: mimicking affinity maturation. *J. Mol. Biol.*, **226**, 889–896.

Hawkins, R.E., Zhu, D., Ovecka, M. *et al.* (1994) Idiotypic vaccination against human B-cell lymphoma. Rescue of variable region gene sequences from biopsy material for assembly as single-chain Fv personal vaccines. *Blood*, **83**, 3279–3288.

Hayden, M.S., Linsley, P.S., Gayle, M.A. *et al.* (1994) Single-chain mono- and bispecific antibody derivatives with novel biological properties and antitumour activity from a COS cell transient expression system. *Ther. Immunol.*, **1**, 3–15.

Herbelin, C., Stephan, J.-L., Donadieu, J. *et al.* (1994) Treatment of steroid-resistant acute graft-versus-host disease with an anti-IL-2-receptor monoclonal antibody (BT563) in children who received T cell-depleted, partially matched, related bone marrow transplants. *Bone Marrow Transpl.*, **13**, 563–569.

Hinman, L.M., Hamann, P.R., Wallace, R., Menendez, A.T., Durr, F.E. and Upeslacis, J. (1993) Preparation and characterization of monoclonal antibody conjugates of the calicheamicins: a novel and potent family of antitumor antibiotics. *Cancer Res.*, **53**, 3336–3342.

Hird, V., Maraveyas, A., Snook, D. *et al.* (1993) Adjuvant therapy of ovarian cancer with radioactive monoclonal antibody. *Br. J. Cancer*, **68**, 403–406.

Hirsch, F., Poncet, P., Freeman, S. *et al.* (1993) Antifection: a new method for targeted gene transfection. *Transplant. Proc.*, **25**, 138–139.

Holliger, P., Prospero, T. and Winter, G. (1993) 'Diabodies': small bivalent and bispecific antibody fragments. *Proc. Natl Acad. Sci. USA*, **90**, 6444–6448.

Holvoet, P., Laroche, Y., Stassen, J.M. *et al.* (1993) Pharmacokinetic and thrombolytic properties of chimeric plasminogen activators consisting of a single-chain Fv fragment of a fibrin-specific antibody fused to single-chain urokinase. *Blood*, **81**, 696–703.

Janda, K.D., Lo, C.-H.L., Li, T., Barbas, C.F.III, Wirsching, P. and Lerner, R.A. (1994) Direct selection for a catalytic mechanism from combinatorial antibody libraries. *Proc. Natl Acad. Sci. USA*, **91**, 2532–2536.

Jespers, L.S., Roberts, A., Mahler, S.M., Winter, G. and Hoogenboom, H.R. (1994) Guiding the selection of human antibodies from phage display repertoires to a single epitope of an antigen. *Biotechnology*, **12**, 899–903.

Kaminski, M.S., Zasadny, K.R., Francis, I.R. *et al.* (1993) Radioimmunotherapy of B-cell lymphoma with [131I]anti-B1 (anti-CD20) antibody. *N. Engl. J. Med.*, **329**, 459–465.

Khawli, L.A., Miller, G.K. and Epstein, A.L. (1994) Effect of seven new vasoactive immunoconjugates on the enhancement of monoclonal antibody uptake in tumors. *Cancer Suppl.*, **73**, 824–831.

Kim, K.J., Li, B., Winer, J. *et al.* (1993) Inhibition of vascular endothelial growth factor-induced angiogenesis suppresses tumour growth *in vivo*. *Nature*, **362**, 841–844.

King, D.J., Turner, A., Farnsworth, A.P.H. *et al.* (1994) Improved tumor targeting with chemically cross-linked recombinant antibody fragments. *Cancer Res.*, **54**, 6176–6185.

Knight, R.J., Kurrle, R., McClain, J. *et al.* (1994) Clinical evaluation of induction immunosuppression with a murine IgG2b monoclonal antibody (BMA031) directed toward the human α/β-T cell receptor. *Transplantation*, **57**, 1581–1588.

Kordower, J.H., Charles, V., Bayer, R. *et al.* (1994) Intravenous administration of a transferrin receptor antibody-nerve growth factor conjugate prevents the degeneration of cholinergic striatal neurons in a model of Huntington disease. *Proc. Natl Acad. Sci. USA*, **91**, 9077–9080.

Kroesen, B.J., Buter, J., Sleijfer, D.Th., *et al.* (1994) Phase 1 study of intravenously applied bispecific antibody in renal cell cancer patients receiving subcutaneous interleukin 2. *Br. J. Cancer*, **70**, 652–661.

Landry, D.W., Zhao, K., Yang, G.X.-Q., Glickman, M. and Georgiadis, T.M. (1993) Antibody-catalyzed degradation of cocaine. *Science*, **259**, 1899–1901.

Levi, M., Sallberg, M., Ruden, U. *et al.* (1993) A complementarity-determining region synthetic peptide acts as a miniantibody and neutralizes human immunodeficiency virus type I *in vitro*. *Proc. Natl Acad. Sci. USA*, **90**, 4374–4378.

Lockwood, C.M., Thiru, S., Isaacs, J.D., Hale, G. and Waldmann, H. (1993) Long-term remission of intractable systemic vasculitis with monoclonal antibody therapy. *Lancet*, **341**, 1620–1622.

Lonberg, N., Taylor, L.D., Harding, F.A. *et al.* (1994) Antigen-specific human antibodies from mice comprising four distinct genetic modifications. *Nature*, **368**, 856–859.

McCloskey, R.V., Straube, R.C., Sanders, C. *et al.* (1994) Treatment of septic shock with human monoclonal antibody HA-1A: a randomized double-blind, placebo-controlled trial. *Ann. Internal Med.*, **121**, 1–5.

Ma, J.K.-C., Hiatt, A., Hein, M. *et al.* (1995) Generation and assembly of secretory antibodies in plants. *Science*, **268**, 716–719.

Mallender, W.D. and Voss, E.W. Jr. (1994) Construction, expression, and activity of a bivalent bispecific single-chain antibody. *J. Biol. Chem.* **269**, 199–206.

Maloney, D.G., Liles, T.M., Czerwinski, D.K. *et al.* (1994) Phase I clinical trial using escalating single-dose infusion of chimeric anti-CD20 monoclonal antibody (IDEC-C2B8) in patients with recurrent B-cell lymphoma. *Blood*, **84**, 2457–2466.

Marks, J.D., Griffiths, A.D., Malmqvist, M., Clackson, T.P., Bye, J.M. and Winter, G. (1992) By-passing immunization: building high affinity antibodies by chain shuffling. *Biotechnology*, **10**, 779–783.

Miller, R.A., Maloney, D.G., Warnke, R. and Levy, R. (1982) Treatment of B-cell lymphoma with monoclonal anti-idiotype antibody. *N. Engl. J. Med.*, **306**, 517–522.

Mittelman, A., Chen, Z.J., Liu, C.C., Hirai, S. and Ferrone, S. (1994) Kinetics of the immune response and regression of metastatic lesions following development of humoral anti-high molecular weight-melanoma associated antigen immunity in three patients with advanced malignant melanoma immunized with mouse antiidiotypic monoclonal antibody MK2-23. *Cancer Res.*, **54**, 415–421.

Moseley, R.P., Papanastassiou, V., Zalutsky, M.R. *et al.* (1992) Immunoreactivity, pharmacokinetics and bone marrow dosimetry of intrathecal radioimmunoconjugates. *Int. J. Cancer*, **52**, 38–43.

Murray, J.L., Cunningham, J.E., Brewer, H. *et al.* (1994) Phase I trial of murine monoclonal antibody 14G2a administered by prolonged intravenous infusion in patients with neuroectodermal tumors. *J. Clin. Oncol.*, **12**, 184–193.

Naito, M., Tsuge, H., Kuroko, C. *et al.* (1993) Enhancement of cellular accumulation of cyclosporine by anti-P-glycoprotein monoclonal antibody MRK-16 and synergistic modulation of multidrug resistance. *J. Nat. Cancer Inst.*, **85**, 311–316.

Newman, R., Alberts, J., Anderson, D. *et al.* (1992) 'Primatization' of recombinant antibodies for immunotherapy of human diseases: a macaque/human chimeric antibody against human CD4. *Biotechnology.* **10**, 1455–1460.

Ortho Multicenter Transplant Study Group (1985) A randomized clinical trial of OKT3 monoclonal antibody for acute rejection of cadaveric renal transplants. *N. Engl. J. Med.*, **313**, 337–342.

Pack, P., Kujau, M., Schroeckh, V., *et al.* (1993) Improved bivalent miniantibodies, with identical avidity as whole antibodies, produced by high cell density fermentation of *Escherichia coli. Biotechnology*, **11**, 1271–1277.

Park, J.W., Hong, K., Carter, P., *et al.* (1995) Development of anti-p185[HER2] immunoliposomes for cancer therapy. *Proc. Natl Acad. Sci.*, USA **92**, 1327–1331.

Pessi, A., Bianchi, E., Crameri, A., Venturini, S., Tramontano, A. and Sollazzo, M. (1993) A designed metal-binding protein with a novel fold. *Nature* **362**, 367–369.

Petersen, B.H., DeHerdt, S.V., Schneck, D.W. and Bumol, T.F. (1991) The human immune response to KS1/4-desacetylvinblastine (LY256787) and KS1/4-desacetylvinblastine hydrazide (LY203728) in single and multiple dose clinical studies. *Cancer Res.*, **51**, 2286–2290.

Press, O.W., Eary, J.F., Appelbaum, F.R. *et al.* (1993) Radiolabeled-antibody therapy of B-cell lymphoma with autologous bone marrow support. *N. Engl. J. Med.*, **329**, 1219–1224.

Riethmüller, G., Schneider-Gädicke, E., Schlimok, G. *et al.* (1994) Randomised trial of monoclonal antibody for adjuvant therapy of resected Dukes' C colorectal carcinoma. *Lancet*, **343**, 1177–1183.

Riva, P., Arista, A., Sturiale, C. *et al.* (1992) Treatment of intracranial human glioblastoma by direct intratumoral administration of ^{131}I-labelled anti-tenascin monoclonal antibody BC-2. *Int. J. Cancer*, **51**, 7–13.

Rodrigues, M.L., Snedecor, B., Chen, C. *et al.* (1993) Engineering Fab′ fragments for efficient F(ab′)₂ formation in *Escherichia coli* and for improved *in vivo* stability. *J. Immunol.*, **151**, 6954–6961.

Roguska, M.A., Pedersen, J.T. Keddy, C.A. *et al.* (1994) Humanization of murine monoclonal antibodies through variable domain resurfacing. *Proc. Natl Acad. Sci. USA*, **91**, 969–973.

Russell, S.J., Hawkins, R.E. and Winter, G. (1993) Retroviral vectors displaying functional antibody fragments. *Nucleic Acids Res.*, **21**, 1081–1085.

Sabzevari, H., Gillies, S.D., Mueller, B.M., Pancook, J.D. and Reisfeld, R.A. (1994) A recombinant antibody–interleukin 2 fusion protein suppresses growth of hepatic human neuroblastoma metastases in severe combined immunodeficiency mice. *Proc. Natl Acad. Sci. USA*, **91**, 9626–9630.

Saragovi, H.U., Fitzpatrick, D., Raktabutr, A., Nakanishi, H., Kahn, M. and Greene, M.I. (1991) Design and synthesis of a mimetic from an antibody complementarity-determining region. *Science*, **253**, 792–795.

Seiter, S., Arch, R., Reber, S. *et al.* (1993) Prevention of tumor metastasis formation by anti-variant CD44. *J. Exp. Med.*, **177**, 443–455.

Shah, M. Foreman, D.M. and Ferguson, M.W.J. (1992) Control of scarring in adult wounds by neutralising antibody to transforming growth factor β. *Lancet*, **339**, 213–214.

Shu, L., Qi, C.-F., Schlom, J. and Kashmiri, S.V.S. (1993) Secretion of a single-gene-encoded immunoglobulin from myeloma cells. *Proc. Natl Acad. Sci. USA*, **90**, 7995–7999.

Slavin-Chiorini, D.C., Horan Hand, P., Kashmiri, S.V.S., Calvo, B., Zaremba, S. and Schlom, J. (1993) Biologic properties of a C_H2 domain-deleted recombinant immunoglobulin. *Int. J. Cancer*, **53**, 97–103.

Smiley, J.A. and Benkovic, S.J. (1994) Selection of catalytic antibodies for a biosynthetic reaction from a combinatorial cDNA library by complementation of an auxotrophic *Escherichia coli*: antibodies for orotate decarboxylation. *Proc. Natl Acad. Sci. USA*, **91**, 8319–8323.

Smith, R.I.F. and Morrison, S.L. (1994) Recombinant polymeric IgG: an approach to engineering more potent antibodies. *Biotechnology*, **12**, 683–688.

Snydman, D.R., Werner, B.G., Dougherty, N.N. *et al.* (1993) Cytomegalovirus immune globulin prophylaxis in liver transplantation: a randomized, double-blind, placebo-controlled trial. *Ann. Int. Med.*, **119**, 984–991.

Stancovski, I, Schindler, D.G., Waks, T., Yarden, Y., Sela, M. and Eshhar Z. (1993) Targeting of T lymphocytes to Neu/HER2-expressing cells using chimeric single chain Fv receptors. *J. Immunol.*, **151**, 6577–6582.

Suitters, A.J., Foulkes, R., Opal, S.M., *et al.* (1994) Differential effect of isotype on efficacy of anti-tumour necrosis factor *alpha* chimeric antibodies in experimental septic shock. *J. Exp. Med.*, **179**, 849–856.

Tao, M.-H. and Levy, R. (1993) Idiotype/granulocyte-macrophage colony-stimulating factor fusion protein as a vaccine for B-cell lymphoma. *Nature*, **362**, 755–758.

Tinubu, S.A., Hakimi, J., Kondas, J.A. *et al.* (1994) Humanized antibody directed to the IL-2 β-chain prolongs primate cardiac allograft survival. *J. Immunol.*, **153**, 4330–4338.

Trail, P.A., Willner, D., Lasch, S.J. *et al.* (1993) Cure of xenografted human carcinomas by BR96-doxorubicin immunoconjugates. *Science*, **261**, 212–215.

Uckun, F.M., Evans, W.E., Forsyth, C.J. *et al.* (1995) Biotherapy of B-cell precursor leukemia by targeting genistein to CD19-associated tyrosine kinases. *Science*, **267**, 886–891.

Valone, F.H., Kaufman, P.A., Guyre, P.M. *et al.* (1995) Phase Ia/Ib trial of bispecific antibody MDX-210 in patients with advanced breast or ovarian cancer that overexpresses the proto-oncogene HER-2/*neu*. *J.Clin.Oncol*, **13**, 2281–2292.

Van der Lubbe, P.A., Reiter, C., Miltenburg, A.M. *et al.* (1994) Treatment of rheumatoid arthritis with a chimeric CD4 monoclonal antibody (cM-T412): immunopharmacological aspects and mechanisms of action. *Scand. J. Immunol.*, **39**, 286–294.

Waldmann, T.A., White, J.D., Goldman, C.K. *et al.* (1993) The interleukin-2 receptor: a target for monoclonal antibody treatment of human T-cell lymphotropic virus I-induced adult T-cell leukemia. *Blood*, **82**, 1701–1712.

Weiner, L.M., Houston, L.L., Huston, J.S. *et al.* (1995) Improving the tumor-selective delivery of single-chain Fv molecules. *Tumor Targeting*, **1**, 51–60.

Yu, Z., Healy, F., Valmori, D., Escobar, P., Corradin, G. and Mach, J.-P. (1994) Peptide-antibody conjugates for tumour therapy: an MHC class II-restricted tetanus toxin peptide coupled to an anti-Ig light chain antibody can induce cytotoxic lysis of a human B-cell lymphoma by specific CD4 T cells. *Int. J. Cancer*, **56**, 244–248.

Zaghouani, H., Anderson, S.A., Sperber, K.E. *et al.* (1995) Induction of antibodies to the human immunodeficiency virus type 1 by immunization of baboons with immunoglobulin molecules carrying the principal neutralizing determinant of the envelope protein. *Proc. Natl Acad Sci.*, USA **92**, 631–635.

Index